Daily Affirmations
For Your Mind, Body & Soul

Jennifer Gagnon

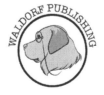

Published by Waldorf Publishing
2140 Hall Johnson Road
#102-345
Grapevine, Texas 76051
www.WaldorfPublishing.com

Daily Affirmations For Your Mind, Body & Soul

ISBN: 978-1-64921-481-2

Library of Congress Control Number: 2020940357

Design by Baris Celik

Affirmations: What Are They and How Do We Use Them to Our Advantage?

Affirmations aren't just meaningless words unless you allow them to be. Affirmations are like mantras—powerful and life changing when used properly. Affirmations and manifestations can bring on a sense of fraud for many. We wonder how the simple act of writing something down or visualizing it can bring it to life, and those that wonder about this aren't totally off. Many try using these techniques without seeing results, and I'll tell you why: You can't write down a sentence or visualize something without meaning it or believing it. If you do, you're getting these concepts all wrong. You see, you have to feel the truth behind them. You have to understand on a deep level that the Universe doesn't speak words, but it speaks frequency. When you say you're beautiful out loud but think how thick your thighs are on the inside, you're sending mixed signals to yourself and the Universe. Same goes with affirmations. You need to say them and mean them. At first, it's hard, really hard, especially when we've been programming our subconscious minds for years with nothing but negativity, fear, and limiting beliefs. Creating new beliefs and thought patterns is not for the faint of heart, but it can be done and pretty quickly I might add. You have to decide. You have to decide you want to create change. You have to commit to the process for however long it takes, knowing that the Universe is right there with you, working to bring your desires into reality. Affirmations are used to shift our mindset and our beliefs. When we say these affirmations out loud, when we write them down with intention, and when we speak those words with determination and certainty, that's when we begin to see the subtle shifts that aren't so subtle at all. In order to make this book work for you, you have to work it. I know you've heard this many times before, but did you do it?

Creating a daily routine that sets us up for success can be nothing but beneficial. It's actually doing it consistently that becomes hard. It has been said and proven that when you're trying to create a new positive habit, it's best to attach it to a daily habit you already have. For instance, if you drink coffee every morning, then make it a point to pull out your affirmations book and do the work while sipping your morning brew. Perhaps you put a sticky note with some affirmations that you need this week on your bathroom mirror and every morning as you brush your teeth, you repeat them in your mind. You see where I'm going with this? Creating a new habit when added to an existing habit allows you to implement new things with more ease. Another thing I want to mention is the feeling behind the words. When you say I'm beautiful or my life is abundant, mean it. Close your eyes and feel how it feels to be beautiful and feel how it feels to be abundant. You might say well I'm not beautiful or abundant, but I call bullshit right there! You ARE beautiful, and if you don't believe that quite yet, then try this: When you close your eyes, how would it feel to look exactly the way you desire to look? Feel that feeling and lean into it with all you've got. If you woke up this morning with a healthy body, all your senses, with a roof over your head, a meal to nourish your body, hot water to shower, and clean water to drink, you are very abundant! Abundance is perception. When you are trying to call in more abundance in your life, you must begin by seeing the abundance that's already there. Close your eyes and feel the feeling of gratitude for all that you have in your life because someone out there is wishing for just that.

When you can't quite wrap your head around the feelings of an affirmation, close your eyes and imagine the affirmation as truth. How does that feel? Lean into this feeling. Using affirmations and daily journal prompts is a great way to start your day. It helps get you in the right frame of mind to create a day of inner peace and freedom. When you allow yourself to step into your powers, when you allow yourself to become the creator of your life, you will be unstoppable. When you are equipped mentally, physically, and emotionally to handle anything that may come your way, then you will experience total freedom!

In the following chapters of this book, I will be sharing daily affirmations that have helped me create a sustainable habit that has done nothing but improve the quality of my life, and I have no doubt it will do the same for you as long as you do the work.

If I may make a suggestion, I'd say don't go further than the day you are on. Choose one affirmation a day to work with and master it. When we are bettering ourselves, we tend to think we need to spend hours upon hours journaling to finally see results, but that couldn't be further from the truth. In fact, I'll go even further and say I'm a firm believer that slow and steady wins the race each and every time. You can't change years of self-sabotage in a day. Allow yourself time to master the art of being fully and unapologetically you.

So, cheers to you for picking up this book and committing to yourself and your growth.

Our minds tend to play tricks on us constantly. We see another beautiful being, and we feel threatened, not because they did something to us but because our self-confidence is so low that we feel less than. We envy our co-worker that seemingly has the perfect relationship because all we see are the seemingly "perfect" bits of her life on Facebook, the highlight reels of her life. We feel guilt for not being able to do it all perfectly because our society has programmed us to believe that in order to succeed, we must be at the top. We feel unworthy because we think that our worth lies in what we own. Releasing these programmings can and will be hard, but if you stick with this book in its entirety, if you commit to yourself first and foremost and do the work, I can promise you that you will see beautiful results.

Simply take a few minutes each and every day to do this work, and you will not be disappointed.

Part 1: Mind

Day 1

I choose calmness where there is turmoil, peace where there is conflict, alignment where there is inquisition, and love where there is fear.

It is easy to get caught up in the chaos that surrounds us. Each and every day the news is creating an epidemic of fear amongst our society. Everywhere we turn we see conflict and war. Remember that you and you alone have the power to choose. You get to shift your focus. You get to shift your perspective, and most importantly, you get to shift your beliefs. Find a positive news outlet, focus on gratitude, and focus on creating inner peace.

Journal Prompt:
How do I get to feel more calmness, peace, alignment, and love in my life?

Day 2

I am whole, I am beautiful, I am loved.

I choose to see the beauty in my flaws.

I choose to feel the softness of my heart.

I choose to sense the divinity of my soul.

When you choose to focus on all that you are and all that you can be, you will be in awe of how far you've come. Focus on the good, so the good gets to get better!

Journal Prompt
Who am I when no one is watching?

Day 3

Life is a dance! I flow with ease and grace, not knowing the next move but open to all possibilities. This is how I experience bliss each day.

Bliss is a feeling, a state of being. Life is a dance, two steps forward and one step back. When you allow yourself to be open to the infinite possibilities available to you, you stop restricting yourself. You stop keeping yourself contained in a box that you've clearly outgrown. When you close your eyes and trust that all is happening for your most benevolent outcome, you allow yourself to dance freely.

Journal Prompt
Where am I not allowing myself to flow in my life? What are the fears or limiting beliefs that are keeping me shackled to this story?

Day 4

I focus on all the things that I can control. My thoughts are pure, my words are kind, my actions come from love, and my reactions are a reflection of the peace I feel within.

When you focus on the only thing that you can control, yourself, you reclaim your power and your voice. When you become aware of your thoughts, words, actions and reactions, you become equipped to face whatever is thrown your way. When you find yourself going down the rabbit hole, you are conscious enough to recognize the trap and pull yourself out of it. When you reclaim control of yourself, you no longer have the need to control others. In this state of being, you reclaim your freedom.

Journal Prompt
What three thoughts that no longer serve me can I release today?

Day 5

I AM SMART!

I AM STRONG!

I AM VIBRANT!

I AM CONFIDENT!

I walk through life with my head high, knowing this is my time to shine!

I AM. These are the two most powerful words you will ever speak. What you choose to say after those words affects you on a subconscious level. The words you've been repeating over and over in your mind over the years have become your truth. Today, you get to create a new truth. One that serves your highest good, one that fuels the wonderful being that you are. Don't you ever forget how special you are. If you weren't special, you wouldn't be here! Do not suppress the thoughts that no longer serve you, rather see them for what they are, old beliefs that you get to reframe. Ask yourself when you began telling yourself these lies, what was happening in your life. Now that you know better, how can you find proof that this old belief is in fact a lie? What is the new belief you get to create for yourself? Write your new beliefs down every day, rewiring our brains can take time, but it is doable and most certainly powerful.

Journal Prompt

What are the lies I've been telling myself? What are the truths on the other side of those lies?

Day 6

I am deeply in love with the person that I am today. I am beautiful inside and out, and I am worthy of my deepest desires.

You are worthy of everything you desire and more. You are unique, you are beautiful, and it is time that you believe these words and feel them to the depths of your being. Know that there is no other like you and that what you bring to the world is needed. You've picked up this book because you are on a path of growth, and you are seeking something different. Step into your power; step into your truth. Feel these words with your heart. Beauty has nothing to do with the way we look physically; our beauty lies in who we are. Love yourself fully and completely here and now. Learn to accept your flaws as they are an intricate part of who you are. You wouldn't be where you are at without the trials and tribulations in your life.

Journal Prompt

What are three things that make me a beautiful being? How do I get to show the world my beauty?

Day 7

I show up each and every day as the best version of myself. I let my heart lead the way to ensure that I never stray.

Live from your heart and less from your mind and ego. The heart will always guide you down the right path. Show up each day knowing that you are doing the best that you can in that very moment with the knowledge and experiences you have. When you find yourself off track, don't beat yourself up, and don't allow your eg to tell you you're not good enough or that you've messed up. Breathe and know that this inner dialogue is coming from fear and old programming. Release it. A good exercise when trying to release old thought patterns is to shift into a new thought. When you catch yourself bringing yourself down, in that moment, edit that thought. Choose a thought that is empowering. For example, if you're thinking something like: " I will never get that position, I don't have the skills", reframe to this "Anything is possible and I am going to learn the skillset I need for this position. If I don't get this one, I'll get one that's even better". Doesn't this make you feel good? When you find yourself thinking "I can't do this, it's too hard", rephrase it "I am capable of anything I set my mind to, I am dedicated to achieving what I set out to and will succeed!". Extend yourself the same grace you would others. Perfection doesn't exist. The only thing that matters is showing up each and every day with the integrity of knowing who you are. Nothing more is required of you.

Journal Prompt
What is my heart guiding me to do right now?

Day 8

I focus on nourishing ME on the inside so that the reflection I get on the outside is exactly that which I desire to see.

When you begin to focus on you and the inner work that you get to do, your outside circumstances quickly fall in line. When you focus on being a better version of you, when you think, say, and do things that are in full integrity with who you are, life on the outside tends to shift accordingly. When you no longer require or expect others, situations, or things to nourish you, you begin to grow and expand. Start nourishing yourself. Treat yourself with the same love and care you do others and see how that feels. When you expect others to fill your cup, you often set yourself up for disappointment. When your inner state is one of peace, your outer state often follows suit.

Journal Prompt
How do I nourish my mind, body, and soul today?

Day 9

I trust and rely on the power of my mind to create a reality I deeply desire. The possibilities available to me are infinite.

When you trust that the Universe has your back, the doors of infinite possibilities open for you. When you trust that you are a powerful being, you know what you are capable of. What you desire is right around the corner on the other side of fear and restriction. Allowing your mind to expand is allowing your world to expand.

Journal Prompt
What are the things that I deeply desire but don't feel worthy of? How do I feel when I think of those desires? How do I reprogram my thoughts around these desires in order to open the doors of possibilities for myself?

Day 10

I live each day fully and intentionally. I show up with ease and grace and simply allow what is to be.

When you constantly try to control the outcome, when you constantly live in a state of fear, scarcity, or lack of, you are missing out on a multitude of experiences. Be present and in the moment. Live your life intentionally by being all there, whatever you are doing. Live fully by not putting off until tomorrow what you can do today. Know that all is happening exactly as it should for you.

Journal Prompt
What do I get to do today that lights me up?

Day 11

I acknowledge my feelings without judgement. I honor myself for feeling them fully and releasing those that no longer serve me with ease and grace.

When you are capable of feeling your feelings fully, you become empowered. This nonsense about only feeling happy feelings is a crock, one that will not serve your highest good in any way, shape, or form. When you bottle your feelings up out of fear or from a place of judgment, you are creating a recipe for disaster. Your feelings are not good or bad, they simply are. Allowing yourself to feel them fully allows you to dig deeper than the surface to find the root of your feelings. These feelings are merely the result of something bigger. Allow the feelings to arise, trust that they are here to teach you something meaningful, and release them. Feeling our feelings is not the problem; living in those feelings and wearing them as a badge of honor is where problems arise.

Journal Prompt

What feelings have I suppressed, and how do I work to release them today? How does it feel?

Day 12

Bliss is the essence of my being. Fear is but an illusion. I show up every day knowing who I am and what I stand for.

Bliss is your birthright. Fear will rob you of it and of so much more if you continue to allow it to. When you allow fear and limiting beliefs to keep you playing small, you are telling the Universe that you aren't strong enough to step into who you truly are. So, stand up and claim what is rightfully yours. You must dig deep and uncover who you are at your core. Know that you are here for a reason, and know that you are capable of anything you set your mind to. Step out of fear and into bliss! Stop allowing fear of the unknown keep you stuck. Fear is merely an illusion created by our minds to keep us playing small. What if you took a chance, you either win or you learn a lesson. Either way, you grow! The more you allow yourself to do this, the more bliss you get to create for yourself.

Journal Prompt
What can I do today that will bring me pure bliss?

Day 13

I am worthy of support, love, abundance, and every-thing else I desire.

Know that you are worthy of your deepest desires. Trust that if the desire arsises within you, it's showing up for a reason. Feel into your desires, feel into the feeling of having already brought those desires to life. Doesn't that feel good? When you believe this to be true, manifesta-tion happens quickly and smoothly. Never allow anyone to make you believe otherwise. The field of possibilities is infinite! What makes you think that your desires are not reasonable? What makes someone else more worthy than you? That's all in your mind. Retrain your mind to know that you too are worthy and that when you begin to believe in the power of your thoughts, the Universe will begin to deliver.

Journal Prompt
How do I feel more supported, loved, and filled with abundance in my life? What do I shift in order to mani-fest this into reality?

Day 14

I allow abundance to flow to me with ease without expectations of when or how because I fully trust that it is already here.

Abundance is in the eye of the beholder. When you truly believe that you are abundant already, you get to call in more abundance. When you are deeply grateful for all that you are and all that you have, the Universe conspires to provide you more of that. When you know you are abundant already, when you are satisfied in the now, you have no expectations about when you will receive more. That is when the flood gates open.

Journal Prompt
What makes me feel abundant right now?

Day 15

I transcend stress, anxiety, and unease. I create a reality that is full of love, peace, and health.

When you no longer allow stress and anxiety to permeate your being, when you no longer make yourself available for the things that create havoc on the inside, you can finally make space for all that fuels and empowers you. Stress and anxiety are the greatest culprits in modern day disease. It eats away at your insides bit by bit, sneaking up on you, and when you least expect it, it will take over your life. Do not allow yourself to get that far. Choose to focus on the now and stop focusing on the past or the future for that is where stress originates from. In every moment of awareness, ask yourself, are my thoughts in this present moment or are they somewhere else? Is this stress I am feeling mine? Is this anxiety validated? Am I stuck in the past or am I worrying about the future? Is this feeling serving me in any way? 99% of the time the answer will be no, trust that you get to be in the here and now. The only thing you can change is your current moment, your current feelings, your current situation. Allow your mind to be calm and at peace.

Journal Prompt

What is causing stress in my life right now? Is the stress I am experiencing going to make this situation better? Does the stress I am allowing to take over my body make me feel good? How do I release this now?

Day 16

I wake up each day with a grateful heart for I am living the life I once dreamed about.

When you wake up each day with a grateful heart for everything there is in life, you create a ripple effect that sends you in an upward spiral of fulfillment. Remember back when you could only dream of living the life you are living now? Be grateful every day for the little and the big things because they all matter the same in the end.

Journal Prompt

What have I taken for granted that I can be grateful for right now?

Day 17

I am a work in progress. I show up today with the knowledge from yesterday ready to learn and grow a little more.

Each and every day you are presented with opportunities to learn and grow. It is always up to you to recognize these opportunities and choose to take them or not. As John C. Maxwell said so well, "Change is inevitable; growth is optional."

Journal Prompt

What did I learn today that will benefit me tomorrow?

Day 18

I take time for me. Time to connect, heal, and grow because I'm worth it. It is not selfish; it is necessary.

All too often we try to be and do everything for everyone around us. We want to be the perfect partner, daughter, mother, and friend all the while forgetting to fill our own cup. We put our needs after everyone else's, and that can take a toll on us. Know that taking time for you isn't selfish; it is necessary for you to be able to show up for yourself and others to the best of your ability. When you continuously run on empty, you are not doing anybody any favors, especially yourself.

Journal Prompt
What can I do today to fill my cup?

Day 19

I take aligned action every day because I am the co-creator of this life. I am magic!

When you commit to creating change in your life, you need to decide, commit, and take action. The only way to succeed at creating something new is to take actions that are aligned with our intentions. You are the co-creator of your life, so make sure that you take inspired and aligned action every day!

Day 20

I ride the waves of life, knowing that after each fall, I will get back up stronger and more determined. The beauty lies in how I choose to rise again.

Know that you can take this life in strides; it doesn't matter if you get knocked down. What matters is that you learn from that experience and you get back up stronger. Know that everything that comes your way is meant for you to learn and grow. Trust the rhythms of your life.

Journal Prompt

What has allowed me to grow that perhaps I couldn't recognize right away?

Day 21

I take in every moment as if it were my last. Appreciating every breath, every sight, every taste, and every experience. This is truly living.

Your life, like that of most, may be running on auto pilot. Wake up, hustle, rinse, and repeat. It's not leaving you enough time to actually breath, let alone the time to appreciate that breath. Take a moment now and pay attention to your breath, for it is your life. Enjoy the abundance of food available to you and eat mindfully, appreciating the multitude of flavors you get to enjoy. BE PRESENT in everything you do. Like many, you take too many little things for granted, and more often than not, those are essentially the big things. When we cannot appreciate all that we have and all that's available to us in this moment, how can we expect the Universe to provide us with anything more?

Journal Prompt

If I were told today that I would not wake up tomorrow, what would be my greatest regret What can I do now to change that?

Day 22

I choose to see life through the eyes of the little girl within me.

When you see things through the eyes of a child, everything brings you to a state of awe: every new smell, every new taste, every new sight, and every new sound. You are easily amused and take most things with a grain of salt. When you look at the world through the eyes of the child within you, you don't see as much negativity, and you don't see as many flaws. You don't judge. You simply live life fully knowing that everything will be ok.

Journal Prompt
What can I do today to release the burdens of my adult life so that you can have fun like a child again?

Day 23

I choose to lead a life filled with fun, laughter, and bliss! Life gets to be exciting!

When you decide to have fun with life, when you make it a point to laugh every day, when you choose to find blissful moments in each day, your life changes. You no longer get stuck in a never-ending downward spiral of stress, negativity, and anxiety because you know how to snap out of it. When you know how to have fun, you not only are taking care of your mind but your body and your spirit, too!

Journal Prompt

What can I do every day to laugh a little more? How can I have fun right now? Recall a blissful memory. Where am I, what am I doing, who am I with?

Day 24

I release attachment to my old stories and programming. Today I stand strong with the knowledge that I am the creator of my reality.

When you release old beliefs and programmings that have been instilled in you for decades, things you "knew" to be true, and when you choose to release fear, you get to create new beliefs and freedoms for yourself fully and authentically. When you are no longer allowing anything outside of you to confine you, that is true freedom.

Journal Prompt

What limiting belief or programming do I get to release right now? What does this allow me the freedom to do or be?

Day 25

I surrender my worries to the Universe, and when I think I'm done, I surrender a little more. I AM all that I AM!

When you allow worries and stress to take over your life, you are giving away your freedom. When you are stressed and anxious, you are no longer living in the moment. You are worried about the past or the future. You have to ask yourself these questions: Will stressing over this issue impact the outcome in any way? Does feeling this anxiety make me feel good? Can I change the past with this anxiety and guilt? More times than not, the answer is no! So why would you allow stress and anxiety to eat away at you, destroying your mind and your body? Choose to catch yourself when stress and anxiety creep up on you, and choose to release it and choose again. Realign and step back into your power.

Journal Prompt

What is something that I typically allow to bring stress into my being? How do I shift out of that?

Day 26

Bliss is the essence of my being. Fear is but an illusion. I show up every day knowing who I am and what I stand for.

When you begin to shift out of fear and into bliss,

you discover this incredible freedom. When you allow yourself to expand rather than be constricted by qualm, you can show up fully and authentically. You can pursue your purpose and truly start living a life aligned.

Journal Prompt

Which fears have held me back for far too long? What would I allow myself to do if I released those fears?

Day 27

I acknowledge my desires and allow them to manifest with ease and grace.

When you are continuously living in a state of fear, a state of limiting beliefs, you are not allowing the things you truly desire to manifest into your life. You are sending a frequency of lack and restriction out into the Universe, creating more of the same for yourself. When you are living your life for others, it's difficult to know what you truly desire. When you want something, you are typically coming from a place of lack, and that is the energy that is output. When you begin to understand what you deeply desire from your soul, then you can begin to manifest with more ease.

Journal Prompt

Where have I been wanting things and coming from a place of lack? What does my soul desire?

Day 28

I dance through the storms of my life, shining so bright that I create my own rainbows.

You can face the things that show up for you with an expansive mindset or a restrictive one. The choice is always yours. Ask yourself a few questions when you are about to go in with restriction and fear. Will this mindset benefit me in any way? Is this reaction of mine going to affect the outcome? Am I showing up as the best version of myself in the way I'm choosing to handle this? Typically, these questions can help bring you back into alignment. They will help you refocus and realign. Then ask yourself, how can I use this experience as a tool for growth? What lessons am I supposed to learn?

Journal Prompt
What "storms" have I experienced that in retrospect have allowed me to grow? How do I get to show up for myself as of this moment?

Day 29

I allow abundance to flow to me with ease and grace without expectations of when or how because I fully trust that it is already here.

Abundance isn't about money. Abundance is in what we experience and who we are. Abundance is waking up each day with fresh air to breathe, clean water to drink, food for nourishment, and freedom to be. Abundance is knowing that you are living your best life in any given moment. Abundance is in the gratitude you feel for all that you have and all that you are. Abundance is being able to move your body in a way that serves you. It's in the laughter you experience and the joy you feel. Abundance is different for each and every one of us, but I encourage you here and now to close your eyes and recognize the many ways you are abundant.

Journal Prompt
How am I abundant right now? How can I create more abundance in my life?

Day 30

I transcend stress, anxiety, and unease. I create a reality where I am abundant in love, inner peace, and health.

Stop spending so much time focusing on all that may be going "wrong" in your life, and start focusing on all that gets to go right. You are the creator of your life, and you need to start taking on that responsibility as if it is the most important one you have because it is. When you allow stress and anxiety to control your thoughts, your words and your actions, you are allowing unease to creep in. Reclaim control now because you can. There is no better feeling than to know you can overcome and transcend anything that no longer serves you.

Journal Prompt
What is causing stress and anxiety in my life right now? How can I release that?

Day 31

Life happens for me and through me. I take each moment for what it is and nothing more or less. I embrace each experience and grow through it.

When you go through life waiting for the next big thing, feeling disappointment each and every time things don't turn out the way you were expecting, you are sending a frequency of lack out into the Universe. When you trust and allow, you tell the Universe that you are ready to receive, however it is deemed appropriate, whenever it is deemed appropriate. When you allow life to happen for you, the outcome will far exceed any expectation you may have had.

Journal Prompt
How have I been restricting myself with my expectations? How can I lean into trust a little more?

Day 32

I AM FREE!

I AM FIERCE!

I AM HAPPY!

When you can live by these statements and carry them with you wherever you go, you will inevitably be living your best life. Imagine waking up each day declaring this to the Universe and actually believing it with every fiber of your being? How would that feel? Change happens when you begin to embody all that you are and when you stand firm in your truth. Declare this loud and clear, and never let anyone or anything mess with this state of being you get to exist in. You are worthy of feeling all of this and more!

Journal Prompt
How do I get to show the Universe that I are free, fierce, and happy today?

Day 33

My life is a series of small miracles. I choose to experience each miracle fully with a grateful heart.

Whether you have stopped to recognize it or not, your life is filled with small miraculous events. You may not see these, but take a deep breath and acknowledge the miracles in your life. As a society, taking things, people, and situations for granted is common ground. Common beliefs that miracles have to be earthshattering in order to be labeled a miracle is nothing but a lie. Today, I invite you to open your eyes and your heart and to witness the miracles in your life: the roof you have over your head, the fact that you wake up each day with the opportunity to choose again, the freedom to make choices, the ability to grow and expand if you choose to do so, the health of your mind and body, the beauty that surrounds you, the changing of the seasons, and life that is created every minute of every day. Start acknowledging the miracles in your life, and I guarantee you will begin to notice more and more.

Journal Prompt

What are some miracles in my life that I can now recognize?

Day 34

I am open to receiving all that will allow me to grow and expand. The myriad of possibilities available to me is thrilling.

You always have a choice in what you believe. Why not choose to believe in the infinite possibilities available to you? Why not live as though everything is possible and waiting for you? Whatever you desire, remember that it's right there waiting for you to have the courage to claim it. You are only restricted by the limits you impose yourself. You are only being held back by the limiting beliefs and fears that you have running in a loop in your mind. Never let anyone or anything rain on your parade. Go after everything you deeply desire and never stop. Allow it all to come to you without expectation. Allow everything to unfold as it should.

Journal Prompt

What have I been holding myself back from? What would I do in this moment if I chose to release my fears and limiting beliefs around this?

Day 35

I allow myself to experience my feelings fully and without judgment. I release those that no longer serve my higher purpose with love.

When you allow yourself to feel your feelings fully, when you choose to stop suppressing those that you qualify as "bad," you begin to heal on an entirely new level. True healing cannot take place until you allow yourself to feel all the feels. Allow them to come to the surface, go within to uncover where these feelings are coming from, and know that no feeling is permanent. No situation is permanent. You can shift at any given moment. Do not judge yourself, simply trust, allow, and release. Let the feelings that no longer serve you go, knowing that they have served their purpose in allowing you to learn and grow.

Journal Prompt

What feelings have I been suppressing out of judgement? What is the lesson I am meant to learn, and how do I get to release these feelings?

Day 36

I am unique. I am a beautiful being, and I love and accept myself exactly as I am. I embrace every part of myself because I am the sum of my flaws and strengths.

Know that you are exactly who you need to be in this moment, flaws and all. Perfection is an illusion sold to us by society. Love yourself as you are now because you are beautiful, you are loved, and you are supported. Stop playing the comparison game. You can't judge a fish by its ability to climb a tree, just as you can't judge your worth based on someone else's opinion. YOU are one of a kind, and you are here to shine bright. The world needs you!

Journal Prompt
How am I unique? What do I love about myself?

Day 37

I see my triggers as opportunities to grow and expand. I allow myself to be shown where work is still required of me.

Triggers are meant to help you grow and expand. You need to dig down into your shadows and shine your light; that is how you overcome your traumas and limit your fears.

Journal Prompt

How can I surrender a little more and learn from myself?

Day 38

I heal my deepest wounds for myself and for all those that have come before and those that will come after me.

We are one! When you choose to heal your wounds, you break the cycle. You can create a ripple effect in the continuum that will heal many. Healing doesn't happen in linear fashion; it happens multidimensionally.

Journal Prompt
What wounds am I still holding onto?

Day 39

I see the beauty that surrounds me, and I see the beauty within me. I take time to indulge in the abundance that is my life.

Your life is abundant if you choose it to be so. What you focus on expands, and when you focus on all that is going right with your life, you no longer have time or energy to focus on the rest. So put a different lens on, and bask in the beauty that is you and everything around you.

Journal Prompt
How am I incredibly abundant today?

Day 40

My reality is a result of my choices. I take responsibility for creating a life I am deeply in love with.

Every choice that you make in every moment will define your current reality. Excuses are what allow you to hide behind your fears, your limiting beliefs, and your anger. If you continuously give away your powers, you will inevitably be living someone else's life. Reclaim control now in this moment, and shift into a reality you no longer need a vacation from.

Journal Prompt
What am I creating into reality in this moment?

Day 41

I create new habits that serve my highest good each and every day. My growth and expansion are limitless.

Creating new habits doesn't have to be hard. One choice at a time, one moment at a time, one action at a time. You get to redefine yourself over and over and over again until you are satisfied with the results. Don't try to do it all at once. Focus on making progress every day.

Journal Prompt
What new habits am I creating right now?

Day 42

My boundaries are firm. I give myself permission to be available to only that which fuels my soul.

Boundaries are necessary for healthy relationships with others and yourself. When you continuously make yourself available to people that no longer serve you, you are leaving no space for those which. Saying no isn't mean or inconsiderate; in fact, it's necessary for your well-being.

Journal Prompt
Where am I not setting firm boundaries in my life?

Day 43

I love myself without condition or expectations. I allow myself to shine bright without fear or shame.

Unconditional love begins with you. Allow yourself to be fully authentic and without limitations. Extend yourself the kind of love you've been seeking your entire life. When you are capable of loving yourself, then you will no longer require it of anyone else.

Journal Prompt
Where am I not loving myself fully?

Day 44

I focus on gratitude, abundance, and unconditional love. I am creating my heaven on earth here and now.

When you put your attention on the abundance in your life and on unconditional love for yourself and others, and begin to live these as your truths, you can create your own corner of paradise. You see, heaven on earth is wherever you create it.

Journal Prompt
How can I focus more on abundance and unconditional love?

Day 44

I am available for my feelings, all of them. I allow everything to surface as it should to be released with love when it no longer serves my highest good.

Too often we tend to suppress our feelings, especially the ones that don't feel so good. The ones we've labeled as "bad" or "inappropriate." It's time to change the current and allow all that is to be without judgement. It's when you allow your feelings to surface fully without holding back that you can seek deeper truth in them. This is when you get to decide if these feelings serve you in any way, shape, or form. If not, you get to let them go with love.

Journal Prompt

What feelings am I not allowing to surface? How do I get to release them with love right now?

Day 45

I AM ABUNDANT! I AM ABUNDANT IN LOVE! I AM ABUNDANT IN LAUGHTER! I AM ABUNDANT IN MEANINGFUL CONVERSATION! I AM ABUNDANT IN EXPERIENCES!

Abundance is in the eye of the beholder. Your abundance may not look the same as your neighbors. When you are capable of seeing abundance in all the little things, suddenly you find yourself calling in more of that into your life. When you feel abundant and know you are abundant, then abundance continues to find you.

Journal Prompt

What are the little things I take for granted that are my true abundances?

Day 46

My boundaries are firm. I give myself permission to be available to only that which fuels my soul

Boundaries are necessary for healthy relationships with others and yourself. When you continuously make yourself available to all that no longer serves you, you are leaving no space for that which does. Saying no is not mean, it is not inconsiderate, in fact it is necessary for your wellbeing.

Journal Prompt
Where am I not setting firm boundaries in my life?

Day 47

Today, I allow my weaknesses to make me stronger and my mistakes to make me wiser. I choose to see all my experiences as an opportunity for growth.

If you keep seeing yourself failing because of one mistake or one shortcoming, you'll never be able to grow into the person you truly want to be. Without failure there would be no success, and without weakness there would be no growth. Focus not on how many times you fall, but on how many times you pick yourself back up and take a few more steps forward.

Journal Prompt
What opportunities for growth have I had recently?

Day 48

My boundaries are firm. I give myself permission to be available to only that which fuels my soul

Boundaries are necessary for healthy relationships with others and yourself. When you continuously make yourself available to all that no longer serves you, you are leaving no space for that which does. Saying no is not mean, it is not inconsiderate, in fact it is necessary for your wellbeing.

Journal Prompt
Where am I not setting firm boundaries in my life?

Day 49

Obstacles are merely stepping stones to something more aligned. The Universe is always serving up what I need.

When you allow yourself to surrender and trust that you are receiving exactly what you need in each and every moment, you can allow all that is to be. You can look at the hurdles in front of you as a learning experiences rather than something you need to change or control.

Journal Prompt:
Where can I surrender a little more? What is holding me back from moving forward with trust?

Day 50

I choose to surround myself with people that are aligned with who I am. I am no longer available for any relationship that doesn't allow me space to grow and expand.

When you surround yourself with people that lift you up and people that love you unconditionally and support you, it's easier to go for your dreams and create a reality you are deeply in love with. Allowing people who bring you down into your life is a choice you make, a choice in which you devalue yourself.

Journal Prompt
Where in my life am I allowing people that are no longer in alignment with me to be in my life? What am I afraid of?

Day 51

I acknowledge my feelings without judgement. I honor myself in feeling them fully and releasing those that no longer serve me with ease and grace.

Feelings aren't good or bad; those are terms that you've been taught. They simply are. You get to choose if these feelings help you grow or keep you stuck. Do not suppress your feelings to make someone else comfortable or because you shouldn't be feeling any kind of way. Just don't allow those feelings to consume or define you. Recognize the feelings when they arise, ask yourself why these feelings are coming up and if they are validated. Once you've gotten to the root of this feeling let it go. Allow your feelings to pass through, just don't keep them over for tea! These feelings that you qualify as bad, are showing up to teach you, to help you grow, to allow you to expand. Take each of these opportunities to dig deeper than the surface, take this opportunity to let go.

Journal Prompt

What feelings keep coming up for me that I suppress? How should I release these feelings today?

Day 52

I choose to embody bliss, gratitude, love, and abundance each and every day. What I create within myself reflects itself on the outside.

Bliss, gratitude, love, and abundance are all choices you get to make each and every moment of every day. It doesn't mean that everything is always perfect, but it does mean that when you find yourself experiencing something that isn't one of those you have the power to choose again.

Journal Prompt:

How can I create more bliss in my life? How do I lean into gratitude each day? What makes me abundant?

Day 53

I transcend stress, anxiety, and fear. I create a reality that is abundant in love, peace, and health.

Each and every moment provides you with choices; some allow you to grow and expand while others keep you confined. Be aware and conscious of what you are choosing.

Journal Prompt
Where in my life am I allowing fear to keep me playing small?

Day 54

I am a work in progress. I show up today with knowledge from yesterday's lessons ready to learn and grow a little more.

You cannot do better if you don't know better. Honor yourself for where you are and how far you've come. Begin to focus on all that you've accomplished to create more of that.

Day 55

I ride the waves of life, knowing that after each fall I get back up stronger and more determined. The beauty lies in how I choose to rise again.

Success isn't about never failing! It's about getting back up after you fall. When you allow yourself to learn a lesson in everything you experience, it is impossible to fail.

Journal Prompt
Where have I been focusing on my failures rather than my wins? What have I done that I am really proud of?

Day 56

I choose to see the wonders of the world through the eyes of the little child within me.

When you allow yourself to see the world through the eyes of the little child within you, you allow yourself to see the wonders that surround you as if you were a child again. Nothing seems complicated, and everything makes you feel abundant. Focus on that abundance, and lean into the deep feelings that come up for you. That's how you can create more magic in your life.

Journal Prompt
What are things that make me feel abundant that I've been taking for granted?

Day 57

I show up every day with a clear mind, an open heart, and a fire within me to step into the best version of me!

When you wake up with a fire inside of you, you get to step into the best version of who you came here to be. When you allow yourself to clear your mind and you open your heart, the possibilities available to you suddenly become clearer.

Journal Prompt
How can I clear my mind and open my heart? How does it feel when I allow myself to do things that I am passionate about?

Day 58

I surrender my worries to the Universe, and when I think I'm finished I surrender a little more.

When you allow your worries to eat away at you, you create havoc within your mind and your body. Worrying about the problem will not solve it! When you ask yourself these questions: Does this worry solve anything? Does this worrying help the situation? Will this worrying solve this issue? What do you get? Most likely the answer to all the above is no, and in that case, why are you allowing it to rob you of your moments? Surrender your worries to the Universe, and trust that all will unfold as it should.

Journal Prompt

How would it feel to surrender my worries and trust that the Universe always has my back?

Day 59

I take actions that are aligned with my intention.

When you decide that you desire change in your life, when you deeply desire something different, you must decide what it is you truly desire and commit to doing whatever it takes for however long it takes. You must take aligned action. This is how you shift into something new and different.

Journal Prompt

How can I start taking aligned action today to create the changes I desire in my life?

Day 60

I love myself unconditionally; therefore, I can extend the same kind of love to others.

Unconditional love is one of the hardest to allow yourself to feel, especially towards yourself. You must understand that until you are capable of giving this kind of love to yourself, you will be unable to give it to others. It's also unlikely that you'll attract this kind of love.

It may be one of the hardest things to do, but it's one of the most rewarding. With one small step at a time, learn to love yourself without conditions, your flaws and all. Each day, remind yourself of how far you've come. Celebrate your wins. Be aware of the challenges that you have and continue to overcome. Acknowledge that you are loveable, always. Love yourself here and now knowing that you are continuously growing and expanding.

Journal Prompt
How would it feel to feel unconditional love for myself?

Day 61

I am no longer a victim of my circumstances. I am the creator of my reality; nothing outside of me dictates what goes on inside of me.

When you allow outside sources to dictate how you feel inside, you are giving your control away. Now is the time to reclaim how you feel about yourself, be loud and proud. Choose to no longer be a victim but rather the creator!

Journal Prompt
Where am I still playing the victim role in my life? In what areas of my life do I give my control away?

Day 62

Today is a gift. I will think, speak, and act all that I desire into reality as I create magic within the Universe.

When you see each day as a gift, a clean slate to choose and create something different, you allow yourself to be the creator. You allow the infinite possibilities available to you to present themselves.

Journal Prompt
What would I do differently right now if I fully trusted that the possibilities available to me were infinite?

Day 63

I AM BLESSED!

I AM LOVED!

I AM HAPPY!

When you allow yourself to focus on the blessings in your life, you don't have as much time to focus on the lack of others. When you focus on all that brings you joy, you no longer focus on all that brings you down. When you focus on how loved you are, you can feel that love deeply.

Journal Prompt
What makes me feel loved, blessed, and happy?

What are the little things that I no longer wish to take for granted?

Day 64

The only time that matters is now because that's all that is guaranteed. I vow to make each moment count and to live authentically, fully, and in integrity.

When you constantly place your attention on what might have been or when you worry about the future, you rob yourself of all your now experiences. Be in the now as often as you can. Appreciate where you are and what you have now. Focus on being fully present because that's where life happens.

Journal Prompt
How do I keep myself from living in the now? How do I choose to shift that?

Day 65

I'm in love with the person looking back at me in the mirror. I am a badass warrior and I honor myself.

Learn to love yourself fully. Learn to see all the wonderful qualities you hold. See your beauty and see your strength. Never let anyone or anything convince you otherwise. You are worthy, so allow yourself to believe that.

Journal Prompt
What are the things I love most about myself?

Day 66

I revel in the abundance that I get to experience each and every day. In gratitude, I create more wealth.

What you focus on expands. Decide to focus on the feeling of gratitude; that's how you call in more abundance into your life. Abundance has nothing to do with money and everything to do with what brings you complete and utter joy.

Journal Prompt
What things or people in your life make you feel abundant?

Day 67

I embody the highest version of the woman I came here to be. I am ready to rise.

Choosing to embody the best version of you means you're deciding to show up as the healthiest, happiest, and most aligned version of you. It takes commitment and determination to rise above the noise. You can always step into something different if you choose to do so.

Journal Prompt

How can I embody the highest version of who I am right now? What choices do I need to make?

Day 68

I am unique. I am a beautiful being, and I love and accept myself exactly as I am. I embrace every part of me because I am the sum of my flaws and my strengths.

Honor the person you are now. You don't need to be more of anything. You simply need to love the person looking back at you. Cherish you and honor you for all that you has been through to get you to this precise moment in time.

Journal Prompt

What have I been through that has allowed me to become the person I am today?

Day 69

I choose happiness, unconditional love, alignment, and freedom. I choose actions that match my intentions.

When you consciously make choices that match your intentions, you never go wrong. When you make choices that bring you joy, when you allow yourself to feel unconditional love and you allow yourself to be free, you get to live your best life.

Journal Prompt
How do I choose to feel today?

Day 70

I focus on inner peace and strength. The state of my inner being allows me to create the most epic reality.

Your outer world is a direct reflection of your inner world. Choose to be aware of what you allow into your mind and body. Choose your thoughts, words, and actions wisely.

Journal Prompt
What can I do today to be more aware of what I'm allowing into my life?

Day 71

I love myself without condition and without expectation. I allow myself to shine bright without fear nor shame.

Show up in the world fully because the world needs your light. Show up authentically and in true integrity with who you are. Those that don't approve were never your people to begin with.

Journal Prompt

What would I allow myself to do and who would I allow myself to be if I let go of my fear of judgement?

Day 72

Today I allow my weaknesses to make me stronger and my mistakes to make me wiser. I choose to see all of my experiences as opportunities for growth.

Decide that you are no longer defined by your mistakes but rather by the way you choose to overcome them and the way you choose to stand back up. Never regret what you've been through because you wouldn't be where you are today if it wasn't for your history, your experiences, your mistakes, and your successes. There is no such thing as failure; you either win or learn.

Journal Prompt

What do I continuously allow to bring me down? How can I use this to grow?

Day 73

I choose kindness where there is turmoil, peace where there is conflict, alignment where there is inquisition, and love where there is fear.

In every moment, you will be presented with an opportunity to make a choice. That choice will either allow you to grow, or it will hold you back. Every single time you are confronted with a choice, choose the higher route; it will always return tenfold.

Journal Prompt
Where in my life am I not choosing the higher route? How do I get to shift that, and how does that make me feel?

Day 74

Life is a dance. I flow with ease and grace, not knowing the next move but open to all possibilities. I experience bliss every day.

When you learn to find your rhythm and allow yourself to be fully guided by the Universe and accept the infinite possibilities available to you, beautiful things happen. You need to surrender the how and when and simply allow.

Journal Prompt
Where in your life are you not allowing flow?

Day 75

I dream as if I am going to live forever, and I live, laugh, and love as if I'm going to die tomorrow!

Choose to live your life fully and happily. Nothing will be handed over on a silver platter; you must be that which you desire and create that which you desire. You didn't come here to hustle, struggle, rinse, and repeat. You came here to grow, to flourish, and to enjoy this experience.

Journal Prompt
How do I create more fun in my life?

Day 76

I focus on the beauty within me and the beauty that surrounds be. I take time to indulge in the abundance that is my life.

When you spend your time and energy focusing on what's missing in your life, you miss amazing opportunities to focus on all that is good in your life. When you take the small things for granted, how can you be sure you'll see the big ones?

Journal Prompt
What do I have now that makes me feel abundant?

Day 77

My reality is the result of my choices. I take full responsibility for creating a life I am deeply in love with.

When you stop playing victim to your circumstances and begin taking full responsibility for your reality, you can choose to do something different. So stop allowing people, situations, and things to dictate who you are and how you feel.

Journal Prompt
Where am I allowing outside circumstances to dictate how I feel? How do I reclaim control?

Day 78

I choose happiness over and over again. Creating bliss in my life by taking one choice at a time is what I do.

When you choose happiness over any other feeling and decide to create bliss in your life because you can, you win!

Journal Prompt
How do I create bliss in my life right now?

Day 79

My talents are infinite. Anything I set my mind to I can and will achieve. I am unstoppable!

Trust and believe that you are talented beyond measure. Trust that you can do whatever you desire because you can. Never allow anyone or anything to deter you from your dreams. Go be the badass that you are!

Journal Prompt
If I fully trusted myself and knew beyond a doubt that I could achieve anything, what would I be doing right now?

Day 80

I approach each challenge in my life with a clear mind and an open heart. I can overcome anything sent my way because I know it's always a great learning experience.

When you begin to take on life as a big learning opportunity, you can only grow. When you begin to see obstacles as stepping-stones to achieving your goals, you come out of each experience better for it.

Journal Prompt
Where in your life are you not allowing yourself to overcome obstacles with ease and grace?

Day 81

I allow my creativity to flow into everything I do. It allows me to express myself fully and authentically.

When you block your creativity, you block everything in your life. Allow your creativity to flow, and allow it to spice up everything you do and everything that you are.

Journal Prompt
How can I be more creative in my life?

Day 82

I trust that I always do the best with the knowledge I have in each and every moment, and I know that that is enough.

When you know and trust that you are doing your best each and every day and show up fully in each and every moment, you must trust that that is enough. When you know more, when you know better, then you can choose to be better. But until then, know that you are enough!

Journal Prompt
Where do I carry guilt for doing something that no longer resonates?

Day 83

I am wealthy beyond my wildest dreams, and the more gratitude I feel the wealthier I become.

Lean into an attitude of gratitude. When you can be grateful for all that is, the Universe conspires to provide more. Don't focus on the things or the words; instead, focus on the feelings. When you are truly and deeply grateful for all that you have, you don't "need" anything more because you feel wealthy with what you have.

Journal Prompt
What do I have in my life right now that makes me feel incredibly wealthy?

Day 84

I have total confidence in who I am. I know my worth and will continue to shine bright regardless of anyone or anything around me.

When you know your worth and show up in integrity with who you are, other opinions of you don't matter. When you know who you are, you no longer need to be anything but you.

Journal Prompt
How can I show up even more in integrity with who I am today?

Day 85

I focus on shifting into positivity every chance I get.

I get to feel good.

When you find yourself in a negative thought, your awareness gives you the opportunity to shift into three positive thoughts right then and there. Every time you are able to do that, you allow yourself to feel good.

Journal Prompt
How often do I find myself in negative thoughts? How can I shift into positivity?

Day 86

I no longer regret yesterday or fear tomorrow. I know that each now moment that I create with ease and grace helps me create the next.

Yesterday is gone, and tomorrow has not come. The only time you have is now, so choose wisely, because your now choice will dictate the next now choice you get to make.

Journal Prompt
Where am I not fully allowing myself to be in the now? How do I change that?

Day 87

I no longer apologize for who I am or what I desire.

I honor my truth; it is the essence of my being.

When you can stop apologizing for who you are or what it is you deeply desire, you can stand strong and unwavering in the truth of who you are. You are exactly where you need to be in this moment, never doubt that.

Journal Prompt
How do I get to show up even more fully and authentically today?

Day 88

I am worthy of receiving unconditional love.

When you are capable of giving unconditional love, you allow others to offer you the same. Love without condition, and love without expectation. It is in this unfolding that you get to be all of you unapologetically; it's how you allow others to do the same.

Journal Prompt
Where am I not allowing myself to love me and others unconditionally?

Day 89

I choose to BE and live in a state of love because love is what I need.

Love is the answer to every question. When you do all things with love, you cannot do wrong. When you choose love over fear over and over again, you allow yourself to win!

Journal Prompt

How can I choose love over fear in my life right now? How does that feel?

Day 90

I AM SUPPORTED.

I AM LOVED.

I AM SAFE.

I AM BLISSFUL

Today I live life fully with no expectations only knowing that all is perfect as it is.

When you feel whole, you become capable of magnificent things. So, trust that you can do today without expectations because the best is yet to come.

Journal Prompt

What makes me feel safe, loved, and supported? How does bliss feel to me?

Day 91

I have the power to create whatever I deeply desire into reality. I choose to do that every day.

When you finally understand that you are the creator of your reality, you will no longer wait for others to provide that which you desire. You will show up fully and create it.

Journal Prompt
Where in my life am I not allowing myself to create exactly that which I desire? How can I release the blocks I am creating for myself?

Day 92

My dedication to myself overflows into my dedication for others. The more work I do for myself, the more I can do for others.

When you continuously pour from an empty cup, eventually you will no longer have anything to pour. Make sure you are fully taking care of you and that you are fully present for you and then you can do the same for others.

Journal Prompt
Where am I putting others needs before my own? What can I do in this moment for me?

Day 93

I do not fail. I learn and I grow. I expand into a deeper awareness of who I am and what I truly desire.

When you refrain from seeing the hurdles in your life as failures, you can grow beyond your wildest dreams. Allow yourself to focus on how much stronger you get back up after each fall, for that is where your power truly lies.

Journal Prompts
When have I gotten back up stronger? Did I honor myself for doing the work?

Day 94

I wake up every day ready to welcome the gifts of the Universe.

When you wake up expecting the unexpected, and allow the Universe to provide you with all the little unexpected gifts, life itself becomes a gift.

Journal Prompts
What small gifts has the Universe provided me? How did it feel to recognize them?

Day 95

I am unique and divine. I am beautiful, and I love and accept myself exactly as I am. I embrace every part of me because I am the sum of my flaws and strengths.

Allow yourself to love you, for exactly who you are, flaws and all. All of you is what makes you unique. The world would be a boring place if we were all the same.

Journal Prompt
What makes me beautiful?

Day 96

I allow my feelings to arise without judgement, for I am not my feelings. I release those that no longer serve me with love, for I appreciate the lesson they are here to teach.

Suppressing your feelings will not serve you. When feelings arise, they are here as a teaching moment. How you choose to deal with them will dictate whether or not you keep repeating the lesson. If the feeling does not serve your highest good, allow yourself to acknowledge it, thank it for showing up, and then release it with love. You are not your feelings; do not allow them to define you.

Journal Prompts
What feelings have I been pushing down rather than dealing with? How does that feel?

Day 97

I choose new thoughts that create new behaviors that in turn create new emotions and new experiences. I choose to grow; I choose to shift that which I desire.

Your thoughts impact your words which impact your actions and your reactions. Everything is energy, and when you desire a different reality, you must choose wisely. Focus on creating an energy you are in alignment with.

Journal Prompt

What thoughts can I create today that will have a beautiful ripple effect on my current reality?

Day 98

I am committed to my health.

I am committed to my happiness.

I am committed to creating a life that I am deeply in love with.

When you commit to becoming the wealthiest person (mind, body, spirit), you will no longer be available for anything that doesn't sustain that.

Journal Prompt

How do I get to create more health and happiness in

my life right now?

Day 99

Today the Universe offers me a blank canvas. I choose to create a colorful masterpiece filled with love and laughter.

Each day is a new opportunity, a new canvas to design exactly what your heart desires. Allow yourself to be creative, allow yourself to trust, and allow yourself to be open to the infinite possibilities and create your dreams.

Journal Prompt
What do I get to do today that will make me feel joy?

Day 100

I embody the highest version of myself today. I think, speak, and take action as the best version of me would.

If you desire something different, then go be that. Stop waiting for the right time; the only time is now. You can be whoever you want to be in this moment.

Journal Prompt

How does the happiest, healthiest, and most aligned version of you show up each and every day?

Day 101

I make a difference in the world by being me, fully, authentically, and in integrity.

The world becomes a better place every day you show up fully. When you are of service to you, you are of service to others.

Journal Prompt
How can I show up fully for myself today?

Day 102

My mind is always expanding. I gain new knowledge every day and that knowledge allows me to be more.

When you allow yourself to absorb new information, you allow yourself to grow. When you know more and know better, you can then do better and be better. Never stop seeking knowledge, for knowledge is a gift.

Journal Prompts
What is something I learned recently? How do I get to be better because of it?

Day 103

I release fear and lean into the Universe with confidence.

When you trust that all is happening in your favor and release fear and expectations, wonderful things can happen.

Journal Prompts
Where in my life am I not trusting that the Universe has my back? Where am I making things more difficult than they really need to be?

Day 104

I am blessed with relationships that allow me to be me and provide me with love and support.

Surround yourself with those that love and support you for who you are, not for this week's version of you. Let go of relationships that do not allow you to grow or to be yourself fully. When you create space, you'll be amazingly surprised at what can happen.

Journal Prompts
What relationships am I in right now that are holding me back? Who in my circle needs me to be someone I'm not?

Day 105

I allow my attitude and confidence to attract amazing opportunities.

When you simply exist in a state of allowing rather than forcing, beautiful things happen. Beautiful opportunities will present themselves to you with more ease.

Journal Prompt
How can I allow more opportunities to enter my life?

Day 106

I am living my best life right now! I am living my life on purpose and with purpose, showing up as the best version of who I came here to be.

When you decide to live your best life now and become unavailable to everything else, that's exactly what you get to create. It's a choice like anything else in life. You get to choose, so what will it be?

Journal Prompts
What does my best life look and feel like? How do I get to create more of that?

Day 107

I am whole. I am beautiful. I am loved.

I choose to see the beauty in my flaws.

I choose to feel the softness of my heart.

I choose to sense the divinity of my soul.

Repeat these while looking at yourself in the mirror. When you begin to believe that these are your truths with every ounce of your being, you'll see your reality begin to change and shift.

Journal Prompt
What beliefs do I need to let go of in order to fully believe that I am loved and supported?

Day 108

I create firm boundaries because I love myself deeply. I am only available for living a life that is true to me and my wellbeing.

Boundaries aren't selfish; they're a necessity. Those that become offended by your new set of boundaries are typically the ones that were benefiting from you having none in the first place. When you begin to respect your boundaries, others will too.

Journal Prompts
Where in my life am I not setting firm enough

boundaries? Who is benefiting from this?

Day 109

I consciously and consistently pivot into a state of bliss.

Change is a choice. Every moment of every day, you have the opportunity to ask yourself if what you are thinking and doing is bringing you closer to that bliss or further away. In that moment, you get to shift or continue down the same path.

Journal Prompt
What truly brings me pure bliss?

Day 110

I allow my inner beauty to shine through fully. I allow myself to express my truth freely and unapologetically.

Your truth is who you are. Never water yourself down to fit into someone else's box. Allow yourself to be fully you regardless of anyone or anything around you. You will be too much for the wrong people; release them and create more space for the ones that appreciate you, the true you.

Journal Prompts

Where in my life am I not being myself fully and authentically? Where am I watering "me" down? How do I change that?

Day 111

Each day I choose mindfulness over worry, love over fear, generosity over greed, health over disease, stillness over chaos, and alignment over discordance.

Every moment of awareness we come into is an opportunity to pivot. If you're not, choose again and make sure you're making choices that are in alignment with your greater good.

Journal Prompt

How does it feel to shift into feelings, thoughts, words, and actions that are in alignment with my deepest desires?

Day 112

I focus on creating more love, laughter, and oneness.

When you focus on creating more of the things you desire into your reality, you have no time left to focus on all that you don't. Always pay attention to what you are focusing on because that's where your energy is going.

Don't forget that whatever you focus your energy on expands.

Journal Prompt
What do you desire more of in your life?

Day 113

I allow life to unfold as it should, releasing the need to control every situation or outcome. I trust my plan.

Releasing attachment to the outcome is one of the hardest things you'll ever have to do. We have a tendency to have a need to control every event in our lives. Remember that when you try to control the outcome, you are closing the field of opportunities. When you trust that the Universe is providing you with exactly what you need in every moment, you open yourself to the infinite possibilities available to you.

Journal Prompt
Where in my life can I release attachment to the outcome in order to open the field of opportunity for myself?

Day 114

My life unfolds in divine fashion as I am guided only by me. I am always open to receive.

When you learn to trust yourself and learn to tune into the powers within, you no longer need anything outside of you for guidance. You must trust that you and you alone have all the answers you've been seeking. Be open to receive them.

Journal Prompt
If I fully trusted that I have the answers within me and trusted that I am a powerful being, what would I do differently?

Day 115

My reality is the result of my choices. I take responsibility for creating a life I am deeply in love with.

You are the creator of your reality. Once you understand this fully and accept that responsibility, you'll begin living accordingly, and you'll make different choices. You'll begin to pay attention to the choices you are making over and over again, and you'll know which ones you need to release.

Journal Prompt
Which choice do I make day after day that no longer serves me?

Day 116

I choose to be fully present in each and every moment. I pay attention to the smells, the sounds, and the beauty that surrounds me. I live not for tomorrow but for today.

Presence is all that we have. Now is all that exists. Lean into each now moment and savor it. Know that you are fully supported, and learn to appreciate all that you are, all that you have, and all that you are surrounded by.

Journal Prompts
Where in my life do I not live in the present moment? What would life be like if I stopped worrying about the past and stressing about the future?

Day 117

I consciously create new habits that serve my highest good. My growth and expansion are limitless.

Creating new habits isn't an easy task, yet it's the most rewarding. When you truly desire to live your best life, you'll take aligned action. If not, you'll make excuses. So, what will it be?

Journal Prompt
What habits could I implement in my day-to-day life to promote wellness?

Day 118

Self-confidence looks good on me as I stand strong and assertive in who I am. I release the need for external approval; only I determine my worth.

The only approval you should be looking for is your own. Your worth will never be determined by someone else's opinion of you. Once you truly know your worth, you will never seek acceptance from anyone but yourself. You are worthy right now as you are! Know that, trust that, believe it with every fiber of your being. Focus on all that you are, and that brings you great pride. Focus on all that you are doing in this moment and celebrate that. In the end, your opinion of you is the only one that truly matters. Every time you find yourself seeking outside acceptance, ask yourself why? Then write down 3 reasons you no longer to seek outside validation.

Journal Prompts

Where in my life do I continuously seek approval outside of myself? Why do I feel I need validation from others?

Day 119

I forgive myself for my shortcomings and all that I did not know. I am committed to doing my best in every moment, and that is enough.

You are not your mistakes. You are the sum of your

experiences and all that you have learned. Know that you have always done the best that you can in each and every moment. If you made a wrong turn, you are not defined by that. You are defined by what you are choosing right now in this moment. You are not your past; you are your now. Continue to show up fully and authentically, and you will never fail; you'll learn, or you'll succeed. Either way you win!

Journal Prompts

What mistakes in my past have I allowed to define me and hold me back? If I believed that my mistakes don't define me, how would my life be different?

Day 120

I revel in the abundance that I get to experience. In gratitude, I create more wealth.

Abundance isn't about money. It's about health, happiness, and alignment. It's about living your best life every day. It's about being aware of the beauty that surrounds you in each and every moment. It's about knowing how to recognize your blessings and to be grateful for them. When you bask in the abundance in your life, you attract more of the same.

Journal Prompts

If abundance is about health, happiness, alignment, and living my best life, how abundant am I? What in my life, right now, makes me abundant?

Day 121

I no longer apologize for who I am or what I desire. I honor my truth; it is the essence of my being.

Stop apologizing for what your soul truly desires. It isn't up for discussion. Honor who you are, honor your truth, and never let anyone lead you astray.

Journal Prompts
How am I not standing in my truth today? Where am I settling?

Day 122

I love myself without condition and without expectation. I allow myself to shine bright without fear nor shame.

Loving yourself unconditionally , you'll allow others to love you with the same level of freedom. When unconditional love is your way of being, you are showing others how you get to be loved. It may be one of the most difficult tasks you'll be handed, but it will undoubtedly be the most rewarding. You are lovable exactly as you are.

Journal Prompt
If I loved myself unconditionally, what would I no longer be available for?

Day 123

I am willing to do what it takes for however long it takes to make my dreams come true.

When you decide to change and commit to doing what it takes, you must be willing to go in for the long haul. Transformations do not happen overnight, and you must be willing to do the work when it's easy but more importantly when it's not. Obstacles will present themselves to you, allowing you to grow and expand.

Journal Prompts
Are my dreams worth the effort? If I fully trusted that all is unfolding for my greatest good, what would I do differently?

Day 124

I focus on inner peace and strength. The state of my inner being allows me to create the most epic reality.

Your external reality is created by your inner reality. When you do the work each and every day, which allows you to exist in a state of inner peace and strength, your reality is a direct reflection of that.

Journal Prompt
What can I do today to create more peace and inner strength in my life?

Day 125

I live in a state of alignment because I decided I am in control of how I feel and who I am; nobody can mess with my vibe.

When you decide that you are unwavering in who you are, you become unstoppable! Choose to live a life aligned, and decide that nobody and nothing gets to shake you. Your vibe is untouchable!

Journal Prompt
If I stood in my truth and claimed loud and clear that I am and will remain in alignment, how would that feel?

Day 126

I choose to be the artist of my life. I will not hand over the brush to anyone else.

You are the artist of your life. The canvas is yours, and in every moment you get a blank canvas to create on. Will you give the brushes to someone else, or will you choose to create a masterpiece?

Journal Prompt
If I fully believed that I was capable of creating my reality on this new canvas, what would I want it to look like?

Day 127

My mind is strong.

My body is healthy.

My spirit is light.

You are all of the above; you must believe it! Look at yourself in the mirror daily and repeat these affirmations. Lean into the truth behind these statements, and lean into the feelings of their truth.

Journal Prompt
How does it feel to be strong, healthy, and light?

Day 128

I give freely and generously as abundance is a gift that gets to be shared.

Generosity is the most amazing gift not only for the receiver but for the giver as well. Nobody ever became poor from giving. Allow yourself to give with love; don't be afraid to share the abundance that you are blessed with. Seek to give not for the validation or applause but for the feeling of joy it brings you.

Journal Prompts
How can you be more generous with the abundance in your life? How would it feel to give more? {It doesn't

have to be money; it can be time, things, a smile, etc.}

Day 129

I see my triggers as an opportunity to evolve. There is no shame in this process; there are only magnificent opportunities that I choose to embrace.

Triggers are just that! You can either fight them, or you can seek their cause. You are always presented with opportunities and life lessons. What you choose to do with them is up to you.

Journal Prompts
What are triggers that have come up for me lately? Why was I triggered?

Day 130

I honor myself on this journey. I have the courage, strength, and trust to go down the path of healing and self-discovery. I am willing to face the darkness in order to find my light.

Honor yourself and your journey. If it were easy, everyone would be doing it. Know that you are always exactly where you need to be. You are continuously peeling back the layers of who you thought you were in order to discover who you were always meant to be, and that is the greatest gift of all.

Journal Prompt
What baggage do you need to let go of?

Day 131

I dive deeper into the depths of who I am every day, discovering new dimensions to explore.

You are a multidimensional being, and you have multiple facets. Allow yourself to dive deep into each one to discover the different levels of your existence.

Journal Prompt
What does it mean to me to be multidimensional?

Day 132

I remember who I came here to be. I live in a deep state of gratitude for all that I am and all that I am becoming.

We all came here with a purpose. We all came here to have certain experiences. Be grateful to be discovering more of that every day you wake up. Accept the gift of self-discovery and remembrance.

Journal Prompt

Who am I truly? Without my labels and personal expectations, who am I?

Day 133

Today I allow my weaknesses to give me strength and my mistakes to deliver wisdom. I choose to seize the moment. I choose to give myself a little grace and allow all that is to be.

Give yourself a little grace on this journey for the work that you are continuously doing for you. Give yourself credit for showing up day after day. Honor yourself for doing the work even if it's messy sometimes. You're doing great; keep moving forward!

Journal Prompts
What mistakes am I dwelling on that I've made in the past? How would life be if I let go of those mistakes and moved on knowing that they made me who I am today?

Day 134

I allow my heart to shine as bright as the stars, allowing the love that emanates to permeate the world around me.

Love always wins! Allow the love within your heart

to be so potent that it can be felt by those around you. Allow yourself to shine bright; the world needs you.

Journal Prompt
How do I feel knowing that the love I emanate truly has an impact on the world around me?

Day 135

I release all limiting beliefs and fears because I know they are an illusion created by my ego to keep me playing small. I am ready to rise.

Thoughts, limiting beliefs, and perpetuating fears are illusions concocted to distort reality. Choose to let go of those beliefs and fears. Trust that all will unfold for your most benevolent outcome, and witness the shifts you will experience in your everyday life.

Journal Prompt
What limiting beliefs have been playing on repeat and holding me back?

Day 136

I show myself the same kind of respect I expect from others. I am kind, I am loved, and I am respected.

When you respect yourself, you open the door for

others to do the same. When you love yourself fully, you show others how to do the same. When you do neither of these things, you set the tone for the way others treat you.

Journal Prompts
How do I truly desire to be treated? Am I allowing myself to be available for anything but that?

Day 137

I am more powerful than my fears, stronger than my weaknesses, and wiser than my mistakes.

Everything that you've been through up until this point in your life has allowed you to learn, grow, and evolve. Never feel guilt or shame around what you perceive as mistakes. Nothing is ever a mistake; it's simply a steppingstone that got you to this place you find yourself in now. You are capable of overcoming anything that does not promote your growth. See everything you experience as an opportunity for expansion.

Journal Prompt
What are the lies I've been telling myself to keep me playing small?

Day 138

The road I choose is one I intend to experience fully, taking my time to enjoy it all because home isn't a destination; it's a space within me.

Enjoying the now moment is the greatest gift we will ever give ourselves. You must trust and believe that now is the only moment that exists. If you aren't living this now moment fully, then are you even living? Appreciate all that is, and know that you are enough in this moment because you are. Trust that you need nothing more than yourself in order to find true joy. You have everything you ever needed within you; you get to tap into all of that regardless of anything else. You are all you need!

Journal Prompt

What would I be doing in this moment if I trusted I needed nothing more?

Day 139

I am wild and free. I enjoy every adventure that nourishes my soul and lights my fire.

Enjoy life because you've only got one! You will never have this moment again, so will you make the most of it? Will you allow yourself to live freely and abundantly? Will you allow yourself to experience all it is you desire to experience, or will you hold yourself back? Will you follow your soul's desires, or will you continue to do the things you think you need to do in order to meet society's standards?

Journal Prompt

What does my soul desire to experience right here, right now?

Day 140

I focus on my inner game because it's the only game.

Our inner narrative is reflected in our outer world. When you focus on what is happening within you, you can dictate what goes on outside of you. When you focus on becoming the best version of you and choose to embody him/her fully and unapologetically, you open the doors to pure magic!

Journal Prompts

Who am I when I'm being fully me? What do I deeply desire? How do I get to be more of me today?

Day 141

I move forward knowing that everything that hurt me didn't break me. It made me the badass warrior that I am today. I honor him/her.

Everything that you've been through up until this moment was exactly what you agreed to experience whether you remember or not. Those experiences are what allowed you to be the version of yourself reading this book. Perhaps some of those experiences are less desirable, but know and trust that everything you've been through was for your own evolution. When you begin to acknowledge your growth and recognize all that you've overcome, you'll be able to recognize the badass warrior within you. You'll honor him/her for all that he/she is, and you'll give him/her permission to keep on shining.

Journal Prompt

If I trusted that all I've been through had a greater purpose and that everything I am currently going through allows me to expand, how would I be approaching every situation in my life differently?

Day 142

Happiness cannot be bought or found on a silver platter. I choose to create it moment-by-moment.

Happiness cannot be handed over; it must be created. You can have all the material objects in the world, but until your happiness comes from within, you will never truly be happy. Happiness looks different for each and every one of us because we're all unique beings with our own unique experiences. What brings you joy is sacred. You don't need to justify what makes you happy; you just need to lean into that feeling every moment of every day.

Journal Prompts

What truly makes me happy? What makes me feel

giddy inside?

Day 143

To just be is the greatest accomplishment of all. I focus on doing less and being more, for my success does not lie in my busyness but rather in stillness.

Being is so much more than doing. Being is the essence of who you are. Your value doesn't increase or decrease with your ability to do more. Your worthiness doesn't depend on how much you do in a given time. Society has engrained this belief that we need to do more and have more to be valued. When you start to recognize the value in being, your world changes. The greatest gift you'll ever give yourself is to just be. Finding yourself will not happen in chaos; it will happen in stillness when you allow yourself to just be.

Journal Prompt
What would I do differently if I trusted that I don't have to do anything? How can I allow myself to *be* more?

Day 144

My relationships are harmonious and uplifting. I surround myself with people who support me and motivate me to be a better me.

All too often we stay in relationships because we think we have to. As we grow and evolve, we must be willing to let go of what no longer serves us, and that includes relationships. You didn't come here to allow others to bring you down. You have to love yourself enough to know when a relationship is no longer serving your highest good. It is not selfish; it is necessary if you desire to continue to grow into the best version of who you came here to be. When you allow others to keep you stuck, you are telling the Universe you don't believe you are worthy of anything different. As difficult as it may be to sever ties, you must know that you cannot call more aligned relationships into your life if you are holding on to those that are not.

Journal Prompts

If I'm completely honest with myself, what relation-ships in my life are no longer serving me? Which rela-tionships feel like a one-way freeway?

Day 145

I always have more than enough. I live a fulfilling life, and I am abundantly wealthy.

When what you have is enough, you are fulfilled. The beauty of this life is that everything you will ever need is within you; everything else is icing on the cake. When you begin to look at how abundant your life is regardless of what you have or don't have, you are the wealthiest person alive. When you feel wealthy, you attract more of the same energy. When you are content with who you are and what you have now, all of it is enough. When you continuously seek more, you exist in a frequency of lack. You are constantly feeling as though there isn't enough. You are programming yourself to believe in scarcity. Feeling that you will never have or achieve what it is you truly desire, feeling as though it's available to everyone but you. Where do you chose to exist?

Journal Prompt
What do I have in my life right now that makes me feel abundant?

Day 146

I am consistently pivoting in order to create a life I am deeply in love with.

You're not a tree, so if there's anything in your life that you are not loving right now, shift and pivot. This is something that you get to do over and over again because you can. In each moment you have a choice, and the choice you make dictates your next. When you find yourself aware of a choice you get to make, ask yourself which choice is most aligned with your desired outcome.

Journal Prompt
If I fully trusted that I was always making the most aligned choice for myself, what would that look like?

Day 147

I am worthy of my deepest desires.

You are worthy of every single desire you have. Make sure your desires come from your soul and not your ego. When you desire something because of what it represents to society, that's ego. When you desire something because you think it will make you more worthy, that is coming from ego. Your soul's desires will feel different. Remember this, the Universe will always provide you with what you desire or something better, so simply trust and allow and know that you are worthy of it all.

Journal Prompts
In this moment, what are my soul's desires?

Day 148

I choose to focus on everything that is going right with the world.

Choosing to focus on all that is going right in no way means that you are only looking through rose-colored glasses. There will always be something that is not going quite as desired; there will always be chaos where chaos is required. Where do you choose to exist? Do you choose chaos or bliss? Do you choose happiness or despair? It IS ALWAYS a choice that you get to make. When you focus on everything that is going right with the world, you make yourself available to see and experience more of that. We all know that your energy goes where your attention goes. Choose wisely where you choose to focus your attention.

Journal Prompt
Where in my life do I need to shift my focus?

Day 149

Whatever I desire I create.

Simple yet so hard sometimes. You get to create whatever you desire into reality. You get to make choices that will call in all that you desire. Sometimes we have to be careful what we wish for though. You must be crystal clear on what it is you desire, and then make yourself unavailable to anything that is not in alignment with that.

Journal Prompt
What do I deeply desire to create into my reality? What choices do I get to make that are in alignment with that?

Day 150

I am grateful for all that I have and know that it is enough.

If you continuously focus on all that you lack and on

all that you want so desperately, you'll forever be chasing something more. When you can deeply appreciate all that you have in the moment and when you become incredibly grateful for everything in your life, you'll truly feel as though that's enough. That doesn't mean you can't strive for something different; it just means that regardless of anything else, you are always grateful for all that you have in the now. Remember when you used to desire exactly this?

Journal Prompt

If I truly believed with every fiber of my being that I have enough in this moment and felt immense gratitude for all that is, how would I feel?

Day 151

Abundance flows to me with ease and grace.

Abundance is in the eye of the beholder, so feel abundant now! You don't need anything more to feel abundant. Waking up today is abundance. Having fresh food to eat whenever you are hungry is abundance. Having clean water to drink is abundance. Having access to all your senses is abundance. The infinite possibilities available to you at any given moment is abundance. So I ask you to take a moment and recognize the abundance that surrounds you.

Journal Prompt

What makes me feel abundant?

Day 152

I am surrounded by amazing people that love me unconditionally and support me in all my endeavors.

Surround yourself with people that lift you up. Surround yourself with people that love you unconditionally and support you in all you do. There's not enough time to waste on those that bring you down. You are worth more than that. You are entitled to feel loved; you are worthy of it.

Journal Prompt
How does it feel to be fully supported and loved by those I surround myself with?

Day 153

I am not my past. I get to create a new narrative, one where I get to thrive.

Your past doesn't define you. It was merely the steppingstone to get you here. Everything you've been through has been a learning experience where you got to grow. Stop focusing on what could have been and focus on what you get to create in this moment. You get to thrive; it's a choice.

Journal Prompt
What would I be doing right now if I truly believed that I could create anything I desire in this precise mo-

ment?

Day 154

I get to change the world one small act of kindness at a time.

The world is changed one small act at a time. When you touch someone's soul because of your kindness, know that you have touched many. The ripple effect is indescribable. Never underestimate it.

Journal Prompt
How can I be of service to others today?

Day 155

Life gets to be easy and fulfilling.

There's this preconceived notion that life must be hard and that we must struggle in order to savor success. Hard doesn't have to mean difficult. It can simply mean that we must put forth the effort. When you do things from a place of love and a place of gratitude, it gets to feel easy.

Journal Prompt
If I truly believed that life gets to be easy and fulfilling, what beliefs would I let go of?

Day 156

I choose to change the thoughts that no longer serve me and replace them with ones that do.

We have over 80,000 thoughts a day, and 95% of those thoughts are the same as yesterday. If you desire something different, you'll have to think, speak, and act differently. When you find yourself in negative thoughts or thoughts that aren't conducive to your growth and expansion, shift in that moment. Rather than focusing on your glass being half empty, focus on how grateful you are to have a glass at all. When you're thinking about how afraid you are of failing, shift into the energy of succeeding and how that feels. Every thought, word, and action is a choice, so choose wisely!

Journal Prompt
What thoughts keep showing up for me that no longer serve me? How do I get to shift into new thoughts?

Day 157

I live in a safe home where I get to be myself.

You get to be all of you wherever you are. Never water down the essence of who you are to make others comfortable. If you cannot be fully you, then who are you really? Are you a stranger to yourself and those around you? Know that it is safe for you to show up fully and authentically. If you don't feel safe doing that, you might want to reconsider how you are living your life? Is it even your life or that of someone you don't even know?

Journal Prompt

Where in my life am I not showing up as all of me to make others feel good? How do I get to change that?

Day 158

The wealthier I feel the wealthier I am.

Everything is energy: what you think, what you speak, what you do, and how you react. The energy we put out is the energy we call in. So, when you feel incredibly wealthy abundant, and grateful, that energy is continuously rippling from you into the Universe, and you call in more of the same. The opposite is also true. Wealth is again in the eye of the beholder, so I ask you to focus on the feeling of wealth and lean into that and watch your energy shift.

Journal Prompt

If I truly felt wealthy, what would I no longer think?

Day 159

I accept myself as I am so that I can accept others as they are.

When we cannot accept ourselves as we are, it is merely impossible to accept others. When we always focus on our flaws and our lacks, that is also reflected in the lens through which we see others. Accept yourself fully, and you will allow yourself to accept others.

Journal Prompt
If I accepted myself fully as I am, how would that feel? What would I allow myself to do?

Day 160

As I declutter my space, I allow myself to declutter my mind.

Clutter around us is a direct reflection of the clutter within us. Look around you and see where perhaps you are allowing clutter to take over. Where are you allowing your mind to feel cluttered? You can purge your thoughts the same way you purge a space.

Journal Prompt
What thoughts keep showing up for me that I need to release?

Day 161

I fully trust the emotions that I get to feel as they are my teachers.

Our emotions are neither good nor bad; those are qualitative words we've learned to use. They are simply as they are. When we can begin to see them as teachers, as lessons, we can begin to grow. When an emotion arises, it's important to allow it to show up fully without judgement and simply see it for what it is. Why is this showing up for you in this moment? Ask yourself if this emotion serves you, and if the answer is no, release it with love, and thank it for showing up for you. Surrender to the Universe, and know that you are now creating space for feelings that do serve you.

Journal Prompt

If I trusted that all emotions simply are and released judgement around them, how would that feel?

Day 162

My natural emotions are love and joy.

We are born with love within us, and joy is our birthright. Don't you forget it! I don't mean any type of bypassing here. What I do mean is that in every moment we can choose love joy. Regardless of anything happening around you, you always get to choose. When you allow everything and everyone around you to dictate how you feel, you're giving your power away!

Journal Prompt

How do I get to experience more love and joy today?

Day 163

I embrace every part of my story, for growth comes with experience.

All too often we feel guilt or shame around our past. Never forget that your past is YOUR story; it's your timeline, and it is that story that has allowed you to become the person you are today. It is those precise experiences that have brought you to this moment in time where you know you get to do things differently. This moment where you know you are in control of your own life. Embrace that because it's what made you YOU!

Journal Prompt
How would it feel if you embraced your story and felt gratitude for all that you've been through, trusting it was exactly what you needed to get to this space you're in now?

Day 164

There are no regrets, only lessons! I either learn or I grow.

Learn to see every experience as a win! You never fail; you either learn or you grow. When you don't see failure but growth, you shift your perspective. It allows you to release fear around failure. It allows you to move forward fully and unapologetically in the direction of your dreams. It's about continuously allowing yourself to continuously move forward.

Journal Prompt
What would I be doing right now if I had no fear of failure? What would be my next endeavor?

Day 165

The better my life gets, the better it gets to be.

This affirmation says it all! The better you feel, the better you get to feel. The more abundant you feel, the more abundance you get to receive. The happier you choose to be, the more joy you call into your life. When you wake up each morning knowing that today is going to be a good day, today will be a good day!

Journal Prompt
What does my best life look like? How do I get to live that life now?

Day 166

I allow myself to embrace the sun in my life as well as the storm.

Our life is the sum of our experiences. Regardless of how you choose to qualify those experiences, they were all put on your path for your own growth and expansion whether or not you can see that right now in this moment. When you embrace every single experience in your life, trusting that you are presented with only that which serves you, you can approach every circumstance with a different state of mind.

Journal Prompt

How can I let go of the preconceived notions I have of my experiences? How do I get to allow my experiences to be learning experiences?

Day 167

I let go of my ego so that I can listen to my soul.

When you clear your mind, declutter, surrender, and allow your soul to step forward, you allow yourself to just be and witness how much you grow. When you let go of ego and begin to listen to the whispers of your soul, you can begin to understand what it is that you truly desire.

Journal Prompt

What would you be doing differently if you were listening to your soul's guidance?

Part 2: Body

Day 168

My body is my temple. One I choose to nourish, love, and respect at every stage and every size; I am enough now!

Right here, right now, YOU ARE ENOUGH, AND YOU ARE WORTHY. Never doubt that. If you desire something different, you'll get there with ease and grace once you learn to love yourself exactly as you are. Desiring more health and fitness is great, but don't forget to love yourself in the process and not only after you achieve your goals because once you reach your current goals, you will already have made new ones!

Journal Prompt
If I loved myself unconditionally as I am now, how would I show up for myself?

Day 169

Every cell of my body is healthy, strong, and thriving. This temple I reside in is pure light.

Your body is auto healing, and when you choose it to be so, you make yourself unavailable for anything less. Your body is your temple, and you get to treat it as such.

Journal Prompt
How would I treat my body differently if I truly believed it was my temple?

Day 170

I focus on nourishing me on the inside, so the reflection I get on the outside is exactly that which I desire.

The way you nourish your body has a huge impact on many things. It affects your internal organs, your brain, and everything else. When you put stress on your body with the foods you fuel it with, you also create brain fog, fatigue, etc. Pay attention to how you are feeling on the inside.

Journal Prompts
How do I feel after I eat or drink? How would I like to feel?

Day 171

I treat my body lovingly, gently, and respectfully. I choose fuel that allows my body to thrive.

Love yourself enough to make healthy nutritional choices. You cannot eat like crap and wish to feel like a million bucks. Listen to your body and what it is telling you. When you feel tired, bloated, or crampy after eating, ask yourself if the foods you just ate are really good for you.

Journal Prompts
How do I feel after I eat? Is this how I want to feel?

Day 172

I embrace the health of my mind, body, and soul. I release all toxicity and choose all that is pure and healthy.

When you put chemically-ridden foods inside of your body, lather chemically-ridden products on your skin, and allow toxicity to enter your mind, all of these contribute to disease. Choose differently. Choose that today forward you will make choices that promote whole health.

Journal Prompt
What can I release right now in this moment that will allow me to be healthier?

Day 173

My physical vehicle is vibrant and healthy. Each day I become fitter and stronger. Health is my wealth.

Health is truly your wealth! Freaking act like it! Your physical vehicle is what allows you to walk, run, see, and hear, and you've most likely been taking that for granted for a long time. Choose to not take it for granted any longer. You get to make choices that allow it to be healthier and fitter every day. So what will you choose?

Journal Prompt
What does it feel like to be the healthiest, strongest version of me? What do I do daily that promotes more

of that?

Day 174

I wake up looking and feeling younger than the day before. I get to experience reverse aging with every choice I make.

Reverse aging is a thing! You get to choose and to believe that you are reverse aging. You need to feel that as your truth with every fiber of your being. Wake up knowing that you look younger.

Journal Prompt
How do I feel when I wake up knowing that I am reverse aging?

Day 175

I fuel my physical vehicle with foods that energize me, nourish me, and revitalize me. I choose health every day.

Food is fuel, and food is medicine. When you learn to live with these truths, you'll make different choices. If you desire to feel energized and good, you'll shift. Today is a great time to choose again.

Journal Prompt

What would I be fueling my body with if I looked at food as fuel and medicine?

Day 176

Optimal health is my birthright, and I affirm that every day. My body is constantly healing and rejuvenating, one cell at a time.

Your body is self-healing. The choices you make will either make it stronger or weaker and healthier or disease ridden. When you load it up on chemicals that do not serve your highest good, you are setting yourself up for sickness. Choose that you get to feel good by eating the right foods for you. When you treat your body with the utmost respect, it will return the favor!

Journal Prompt
What does it feel like to be living in a body that is extremely healthy and strong?

Day 177

I love the reflection looking back at me in the mirror.

Love yourself exactly as you are. You are beautiful, you are unique, you are strong, and you are healthy. Treat your body well because you love it, move it because you love it, and respect it because you love it.

Journal Prompt

How does it feel when I love myself exactly how I am?

Day 178

As I breathe deeply, I fill my lungs with pure energy. Sending a wave of healing through my body, restoring every cell, every molecule, and removing all that is not in my highest good.

Breath is life. Pay attention to the way you breathe, and choose to regulate it. All too often you don't pay attention to your breath because it's one of those things that just happens. Be aware of your breath; it says a lot about what is happening within you. Slow down, regulate, and choose to breathe in life and exhale stress.

Journal Prompt

How does it feel to know that I have the tools to heal; mind, body & spirit?

Day 179

My body is radiant.

My body is strong.

My body is fit.

Our body is intricate; it is made up of multiple systems and organs, and it is truly amazing. Learn to pay attention, and learn to be grateful for this body you were given. It is unique because you are unique. Love yourself as you are even if you're striving for change.

Journal Prompt
How does it feel to be strong, radiant, and fit? What feelings come up when I read this sentence?

Day 180

I listen to my body now, so I don't have to suffer the pain of its shrieks later.

Your body is constantly giving you subtle signs in hopes you'll listen. When you are not in tune with yourself and you simply are in the habit of going through the motions, you'll often miss those signs. Know that if you continue to ignore them, sooner or later your body will have to take radical action for you to pay attention. All too often that appears in the form of disease, pain, etc. Tune into you; learn to feel where there may be tension or subtle pain. The better you get at listening, the quicker you can shift and pivot to remedy any situation.

Journal Prompt
How does it feel to know that I am in tune with my body?

Day 181

Every cell of my body is thriving. I am healthier and feel more and more restored each and every day.

Your body is always repairing, healing, and doing some pretty incredible stuff you know nothing about. When your body is doing exactly what you want it to and feel "fine," you don't realize how hard your body is working for you. Honor and thank it for allowing you to do all that you do.

Journal Prompt
How do I get to help my body restore and repair itself with more ease?

Day 182

I wake up energized, bright eyed, and ready to take on the day.

When you care for yourself in a manner that enhances your health, you'll wake up energized and ready to take on the day. If not, that's a great indicator that perhaps you need to shift certain habits. Creating daily routines that allow our bodies to function optimally is one of the greatest gifts.

Journal Prompt
What can I do today to feel even better than yesterday?

Day 183

I choose to move my body to help it heal, strengthen, and thrive.

Move your body because you love it, not to punish it. Movement is extremely important for your muscles, your joints, your mindset, and your energy. It's important for every part of you. Movement doesn't have to look a certain way. Find a way that brings you joy. Move in a way that allows you to feel free and happy.

Journal Prompt
How does it feel to move my body, knowing that I am doing something good for me?

Day 184

My health is my wealth and my priority. Every choice I make creates more of that.

Every choice you make every day either promotes health or disease. Be sure to make choices that are in alignment with what it is you desire.

Journal Prompt
What choices did you make today that promoted a healthy body?

Day 185

I create balance in my body by listening to what it needs. It always knows best.

Your body speaks to you in not so many words. The little nudges you feel, the bloating, the lack of energy, the fatigue, the brain fog, the irritability, and the negative thoughts, there to nudge you in another direction. You aren't supposed to feel exhausted all the time, and you're not supposed to feel irritable all the time. When you slow down and begin to listen, you'll be able to decipher what it is you get to do differently.

Journal Prompt
What are some subtle signs my body has been sending me that perhaps I wasn't paying attention to?

Day 186

I am not my hair.

I am not my size.

I am not the number on a scale.

You are none of those things. Your external appearance does not define you. What defines you is who you are at your core. Health has nothing to do with a size or a number on a scale; it has to do with how you feel.

Journal Prompt
If you loved your body exactly how it is now, what would you stop telling yourself?

Day 187

My body heals quickly and effectively.

Our body is always working, always healing. Honor its work, and honor how far it has carried you. Honor the magic it can create. Be grateful for its strength; be grateful for all it has done for you thus far.

Day 188

I move my body daily in a way that feels good.

Move every day, not because you have to or because you hate your body but because you love it and because it can. Find something that brings you joy and brings on a sweat and do that!

Journal Prompt
What makes me feel really good? How do I get to incorporate more of that into my life?

Day 189

I workout because I love my body and because my body loves me.

Love your body, and it will love you back. Never underestimate its capabilities and how hard it works. Trust it and create an environment where it can thrive.

Journal Prompt
What can I do today to love my body a little more?

Day 190

I am grateful for my senses. They are a gift not given to all.

Have you ever stopped to think what life would be like if you woke up tomorrow without your senses? Like many, you probably haven't. Your senses allow you to see the beauties that surround you, to hear the sweet melody of children's laughter, and to feel the softness of a touch. If you've taken them for granted, in this moment, revel in gratitude for all that you have available to you.

Journal Prompt
How incredible is life thanks to your senses?

Day 191

This body of mine is the only one I get. I choose to

honor and respect it.

Every day is a new opportunity to become healthier. Nourish your body with healthy foods, move a little, choose thoughts that allow you to grow and feel your best, take actions to fill your cup, make choices that reduce stress, find joy in each experience.

Journal Prompt
What do I get to do today that will create more health within my vessel?

Day 192

I am always learning. My mind is a beautiful mechanism that allows me to learn anything I desire.

Your mind is your greatest asset. You can use it to your advantage each and every day. Anything you desire to learn is possible if you take the necessary steps.

Journal Prompt
If I trusted that the possibilities available to me were infinite, what would I be doing right now?

Day 193

I AM BEAUTIFUL.

I AM UNIQUE.

I AM SPECIAL

You are all of those things Trust that you are beautiful as you are. You are unique and you are special, never let anyone or anything make you doubt that. Feel the energy behind those words and trust that with all that you are.

Journal Prompt
What are my most amazing qualities?

Day 194

I send love and light to every cell of my body, every molecule of my being. I am allowing it to heal and release what no longer serves it now.

You are a powerful being, and you get to heal yourself if you choose to do so. When you trust yourself enough to release all that no longer serves you, you create space to call in all that does.

Journal Prompt

What do I get to release today that no longer serves my body?

Day 195

I love my body exactly the way it is and continue to allow it to expand into more health.

Love yourself fully as you are. No holdbacks, no "I'll love myself when." LOVE YOURSELF NOW!! Treat yourself with respect and demand the same of others. Celebrate you, all of you. Stop waiting for to have the perfect hair, the perfect skin, the perfect weight… know that you are perfectly imperfect now and embrace all that you are. Speak to yourself kindly and gently. Show yourself a little extra grace when you feel like giving up. Treat your body with love. Allow yourself to expand into more health and wellness.

Journal Prompts
How can you love yourself more today? What does that look like?

Day 196

I honor my physical vehicle as it allows me the privilege to run, walk, dance, smell, see, and hear. This body of mine is pretty rad.

Your body is freaking rad, so treat it as such!

Journal Prompt
If I truly believed that my body is the greatest gift ever, what would I be doing to take care of it now?

Day 197

I deserve to love the body I have.

Your body does not need to be a certain way; it needs to be exactly as it is. It needs you to love it and nourish it. That's what it needs first and foremost!

Journal Prompt
What beliefs do I need to let go of in order to love myself fully?

Day 198

Every day I feel more and more comfortable in my own skin, appreciating all that I am now.

You get to choose every day to honor yourself where you're at. You get to love the person you are, inside and out.

Journal Prompt
What can I do today to feel even more in love with who I am?

Day 199

With every workout, my body builds itself a little stronger.

Day 200

I choose to move my body today to allow my energy to flow easily and abundantly.

When you move your body, you allow the energy to flow. When you are continuously living a sedentary life, the energy becomes stagnant and all areas of your life are affected. Choose to move!

Journal Prompt
How do I get to move today that will allow me to feel good?

Day 201

The more flexible my body becomes, the more flexible my mind becomes. It's a harmony that I choose to create.

Our bodies are incredibly capable beyond what our minds can imagine. You can do whatever you desire. Your body remembers what you've been doing, and as with anything else, the more you do something, the better you become at it. When you realize the extent of what your body can do, you also stretch your mind to see what it can also do.

Journal Prompt
If I trusted my body can truly do whatever I desire, what would I try that I haven't allowed myself to?

Day 202

Moving my body is my therapy. It allows me to get out of my mind and into my body, creating a deep connection to my senses.

Moving your body will allow you to let go of all the tension you've been holding onto. See your movement sessions as more than what meets the eye because they are. They don't only allow your body to strengthen, they allow your mind to get clear and your energy to flow.

Journal Prompt

How do I feel after I've moved my body in a way that feels good?

Day 203

I choose to thrive physically, for it allows me to also thrive mentally and spiritually.

All areas of our life are intertwined and interconnected, and when you choose to work on one area, it will inevitably affect all others. See yourself as the whole being that you are. You are not just your body, you are not just your mind, and you are not just your soul. You are a sum of all of that.

Journal Prompt

What can I choose in this moment that will allow me to get closer to my goals?

Day 204

Every step I take towards greater health allows my body to heal a little more.

Every choice you make either allows you to heal a little more or not. It is always up to you.

Journal Prompt

What can I do right now in this moment that will make me healthier?

Day 205

I am deeply in love with the body I have. It has allowed me to bring the greatest miracles into this world.

Your body has allowed you to do all that you've done and will allow you to do all the things you deeply desire to do. Honor that and stop taking it for granted. Your healthy body allows you to help others, to give birth, and to care for others; it allows you to create so many miracles. Never underestimate its worth.

Journal Prompt

What is something your healthy body allowed you to do that you are incredibly proud of in retrospect?

Day 206

My body has the power to heal itself. I get to assist the healing with each choice I make.

Your body is an auto healing machine; you can either contribute to the optimal functioning of it or to its demise. The choice is always yours. Reclaim control of your health because you can.

Journal Prompt
What does optimal health feel like?

Day 207

I'm grateful for my senses. It is a great gift to be able to see the trees, hear the birds, taste the nectar, and feel the wind.

When you become capable of recognizing the simple gifts of life, you can begin to recognize that they are in fact the big ones. So many things we take for granted that ARE in reality our greatest gifts. Never doubt that.

Journal Prompt
What have I taken for granted in the past that I am deeply grateful for?

Day 208

I choose gratitude each and every day for the ability

to do better than yesterday.

Every day, you have the opportunity to repeat history or create something new. Do you see each day as a clean slate or the continuance of the day before? Each day, you get to choose again. You get to choose a different narrative, one that is aligned with who you are.

Journal Prompt
If I believed that I get to choose again, what would I choose today?

Day 209

When I move with more freedom and flow, life gets to be a party.

Learn to move with ease and flow. Life truly is a dance, and you get to choose your next move. Stop following the beat of those around you, and choose to create your own rhythm.

Journal Prompt
How do I get to move today in a way that makes me feel abundant?

Day 210

I allow my inner beauty to shine through fully. I allow myself to express my truth freely and unapologetically.

Stop playing small to make others feel comfortable. Stop watering yourself down in order to fit in. You were born unique and beautiful; you were made to stand out.

Journal Prompt
Where in my life have I not allowed myself to be myself fully? How can I change that in this moment?

Day 211

I feel more vibrant and energized with every choice I make. I am consistently maintaining a healthy temple.

When you feel depleted and exhausted, you are of no service to yourself nor others. When you make choices that light you up and invigorate you, you show up fully for yourself and others. Why would you knowingly choose anything but that?

Journal Prompt
When do I feel most energized and invigorated? How do I get to feel that energy more and more?

Day 212

Happiness is a choice that I make constantly. I am

infinitely abundant, and for that I am grateful.

Happiness is homemade. You've heard it before, but have you truly taken on that responsibility? It's easy to play victim and put the blame on others. Nobody can make you unhappy unless you allow them to, so reclaim control here and now because you can.

Journal Prompts
What truly makes me happy? How can I create more of that in my life?

Day 213

I heal on a cellular level every day. My mind, my body, and my spirit are on a constant path of transformation and transmutation.

Your body desires to heal, and your body has the capability of restoring itself if you allow it to be. Be wise in the choices that you make, and be aware of the outcome you desire.

Journal Prompt
How do I get to allow my body to heal a little more today?

Day 214

I am deeply in love with this life that I get to live. Every moment gets to feel magical and fulfilling.

Your life gets to feel magical if you allow it to be. Each moment is magic: the fact that you are breathing, the fact that you have the freedom to choose again, and the fact that your body allows you to move in all the ways you can think of. When you see magic, you become magic.

Journal Prompt
How do I get to create more magic in my life right now?

Day 215

I allow myself to be amazed by life and its infinite beauty. Like a child, without expectation nor judgement I can receive freely.

When you allow yourself to be in awe of all that is and look at life through the eyes of a child, everything is wonderful and amazing. When you have no expectations or judgement and truly know with every fiber of your being that you are always being presented with something more marvelous than the last, you begin to live freely and abundantly.

Journal Prompt
What beauties am I surrounded by right now?

Day 216

I allow love to permeate everything that I am and everything that I do. In this state of being, I am free.

Love is where it began, and love is where it ends. Love is the ultimate emotion. When you love unconditionally, you free yourself from the shackles of anger, jealousy, hate, and all those feelings that no longer serve you. When you become capable of existing in a state of love, you become free!

Journal Prompt
If I truly existed with unconditional love for myself, what would I be doing differently?

Day 217

I allow myself to slow down. I allow myself to find the answers to my deepest inquiries in stillness.

In this life we've created for ourselves, all too often we are perpetually entering the rat race. We seek more success, more money, and more material things. Give yourself permission to slow down, and allow yourself to be still and just be. Only in stillness and silence can you allow yourself to listen to the whispers within.

Journal Prompt
What are my beliefs around stillness?

Day 218

I am grateful for this body I have been blessed with. It is healthy, vibrant, and all its cells work in perfect harmony.

Your body is unique, and it is yours. It is a beautiful work of art, and you get to treat is as such. Allow it to work for you by giving it all it needs. Love and respect yourself enough to care. Give yourself permission to do things that make you feel good.

Journal Prompt
How have I been self-sabotaging myself in the past? How do I get to shift out of that today?

Day 219

My body is healthy.

My mind is clear.

My soul is pure.

I manifest paradise right here, right now.

When you tune into you and become in alignment with who you are at your core, magic happens. When you are continuously shifting and pivoting in the direction of your desires, you allow yourself to manifest YOUR paradise on earth. You create the reality you never need a vacation from.

Journal Prompt

What does paradise on earth look and feel like for me?

Day 220

Healing energies flow freely and abundantly through my entire being. I am left with a clear mind, a vibrant body, and a tranquil soul.

Healing energies are abundantly available to you if you allow them to be. When you open yourself to only the energies that are there for your most benevolent outcome, you allow them to pour through your entire being and do their thing.

Journal Prompt

Where in my life am I blocking my own healing?

Day 221

My body is my temple; it is my shrine. I focus on giving it nothing but the best physically, mentally, emotionally, and spiritually.

Your body is truly your temple! It's the only place you have to live; you only have one body! If you do not treat it well and put its well-being first and it fails you, what will you do? Choose to take care of it as if you could never get another one because you can't!

Journal Prompt
How can I treat my being like the temple that it is?

Day 222

My vessel is my temple. I release toxicity from my mind, body, spirit, and environment in order for it to thrive.

When you love yourself enough to care, you can begin to take inventory and see where you are allowing toxicity to seep in. Toxins come in many shapes and sizes. Some are seen and others unseen. Decide to remove toxicity from your environment, from your foods, from your beauty products, from your cleaning products, from your mind, from your circle, and from every area of your life. When you release toxicity, you make space for all the things that will allow you to grow, heal, and expand.

Journal Prompts
Where am I allowing toxicity in my life? How do I get to release all of that?

Day 223

My body is a sacred temple of love and light, and I treat it as such.

When you love yourself enough to care, you can begin to take inventory and see where you are allowing toxicity to seep in. Toxins come in many shapes and sizes. Some are seen and others unseen. Decide to remove toxicity from your environment, from your foods, from your beauty products, from your cleaning products, from your mind, from your circle, from every area of your life. When you release toxicity, you make space for all the things that will allow you to grow, heal and expand.

Journal Prompt
Where am I allowing toxicity in my life? How do I get to release all of that?

Day 224

I am constantly amazed at the strength of my body and all it can do.

Your body is so strong even when you treat it poorly. Your body gets put through the wringer every day, yet it always shows up for you. Take a minute to see all that your body is and all that it does and sit with your feeling of gratitude.

Journal Prompt
How did my body show strength today?

Day 225

I create perfect harmony within my body. My organs and systems work in symphony together, creating whole health.

Creating balance in your being also creates harmony. When you create a sacred space within you and treat your being as the beautiful kingdom that it is, it will reward you tenfold. Allow your systems to function optimally with every decision you make.

Journal Prompt
How can I create more health within my being today?

Day 226

I release tensions and aches from my body because they do not serve me. I create space for more healing and well-being within me.

Allow yourself to release any tension and pain. Know that they no longer serve you. Utilize the tools available to you that will help you feel good.

Journal Prompts
Where am I carrying tension and pain in my body? How do I get to let that go?

Day 227

Positive and healing energies flow through my entire being, leaving health in its path.

Healing energies are everywhere; will you allow them in? Choose to believe that you are capable of healing every cell in your being. Feel the feeling of that healing, and lean into it. When you can feel the feeling even before the event occurs, you become your own healer.

Journal Prompt
What am I allowing myself to heal?

Day 228

I am proud of the work that I do each and every day to be the healthiest I can be.

Be proud of all that you do for you. Show up for yourself and give yourself credit for how far you've come. Each little step in the right direction over time adds up to a massive change. The compound effect is real, and you should celebrate yourself every day for what you are accomplishing.

Journal Prompt
Where am I not giving myself enough credit for all that I've done and continue to do?

Day 229

I am grateful that my body knows exactly what to do to heal and restore itself.

Be grateful that your body knows what to do. Be grateful that however you've chosen to treat your body up until this point, it has continued to show up for you. Know that it will continue to show up for you.

Journal Prompts

What choices do I keep making that don't promote health? How do I get to choose something different?

Day 230

My body allows me to move effortlessly and swiftly.

Focus on how good your body feels, and focus on how well it moves. Recognize the beauty of all that you are. You wake up each morning without having to think about getting up or walking; your body just does. You do not need to think about breathing; you just do. You don't have to think about opening your eyes; you just do. Your body is functioning beautifully and effortlessly.

Journal Prompt

What did my body allow me to do today?

Day 231

My cells regenerate themselves continuously, leaving my being refreshed and restored.

Your cells are rejuvenating and regenerating every second of every day. You don't see all the work that's happening within your body, but that doesn't mean it's not happening. You get to wake up refreshed and invigorated each and every day!

Journal Prompt
How does my body feel when I'm energized?

Day 232

I use food to fuel my body and allow it to get stronger and fitter.

Food is fuel, so choose what you put in your body wisely. You can't feed yourself items from the dollar menu and expect to feel like a million bucks. You get to choose differently because you desire to be healthier, fitter, and stronger.

Journal Prompt
If there was a window to your stomach and everyone could see what you put in your body, would you walk proudly, or would you want to hide?

Day 233

This fully functioning body of mine is a gift I will no longer take for granted. I appreciate everything it has gotten me through.

Never take who you are for granted. Never take what you are capable of for granted. Your worthiness does not come from someone else's opinion of you; it comes from YOU!

Journal Prompt
If I truly believed I was worthy, how would I be treating myself every day?

Day 234

I trust my body is exactly as it needs to be in this moment. I will continue to love it as I help it become stronger and fitter.

Your body is exactly where it needs to be in this moment. If you're striving for something different, that's okay. You need to learn to love every single phase of your body. Love yourself every step of the way because you deserve it!

Journal Prompt
If you loved yourself unconditionally at every stage of your journey, how would you speak to yourself?

Day 235

I eat intuitively and listen to what my body is asking for.

Listen to what your body is telling you; it knows best. Oftentimes we eat and feel crappy. We feel tired, bloated, etc. Pay attention! You're getting all the signs, but if you're not paying attention, you won't notice them. Any discomfort is abnormal. See what foods you are eating that aren't agreeing with you.

Journal Prompts
What foods make me feel amazing? What foods make me feel tired, moody, or bloated?

Day 236

I breathe consciously and with intention to allow my body to heal.

Breath is life. Pay attention to your breath; it has a lot to show you. Slowly breathe in life and exhale all the bullshit you've been keeping in. Allow your breath to become not only your lifeline but the mechanism with which you get to release your stress and anxiety.

Journal Prompts
When I pay attention to my breath, is it fast, shallow, deep, or restorative? Now breathe in for 5 seconds, hold at the top for 5 seconds and exhale for 5 seconds. How

did that feel?

Day 237

My sleep is deep and restorative. I wake up ready to hit the ground running.

Sleep is so important, yet so many people are running on fumes. So many people will skip sleep and not realize the amount of stress it puts on their body and mind. Make sure that you are waking up feeling refreshed and ready to take on the day. Don't run on fumes. It'll catch up with you, and it will affect your health.

Journal Prompt
How do I feel when I wake up in the morning?

Day 238

I am in perfect health, and my body is functioning optimally.

Make sure that you are contributing to its health and expansion.

Journal Prompt
What do you get to do when you are abundantly healthy?

Day 239

I am patient with myself, and I allow myself time to create the body I feel good in.

Be patient with yourself. Know that you are doing the best you can with the information you have in this precise moment. The more you know the more you get to do. Focus on all you've accomplished and then move forward from there.

Journal Prompt
What do you get to do today that will get you closer to your health goals?

Day 240

I take consistent aligned action every day in order to feel the way I desire to feel.

You get to feel however you choose to feel. You get to create whatever you choose to create. You simply need to decide, commit, and take aligned action. That's truly all that's required.

Journal Prompts
What does taking aligned action look like for you? Have you been taking aligned action, or have you been finding excuses?

Day 241

I choose health & happiness every day.

Health is a choice, just like everything else in your life. Every decision you make either promotes health or disease. The foods you choose to fuel your body with, the thoughts you feed your mind, the feelings you choose to entertain, the limiting beliefs you hold onto, all of these dictate how healthy or unhealthy you get to be. What are you choosing?

Journal Prompt
If you look at the choices you've made this week, did they promote health or disease?

Day 242

My immune system is strong and ready to fight. I help strengthen it with every choice I make.

Your immune system is always ready to fight for you. It is one of your greatest allies, and it will go to war against disease for you. You get to help it function optimally each day with everything you put in and on your body. Pay attention to all that you are allowing to enter your body.

Journal Prompt
What would you be doing differently if you were to focus on boosting your immune system?

Day 243

My nervous system gets to rest as I find stillness and create a safe space for myself.

Your nervous system is intricate and important. Pay attention to what you're currently doing and if it's beneficial to you or not. You are in charge of all of your systems; each choice you make either strengthens them or weakens them.

Journal Prompt

What would you do differently if you knew you could feel amazing every day?

Day 244

I am beautiful and strong just the way I am.

You are beautiful exactly as you are. Comparison is the biggest thief of joy; don't fall into the trap. You are exactly as you should be, or else you wouldn't be the way you are! You are unique and special. Don't ever let anything or anyone convince you otherwise.

Journal Prompt

If I truly believed I am beautiful, how would I show up in the world?

Day 245

I am proud of how far I've come and the work that I've done. My body is mine, and I continue to strengthen it.

Feel pride for all that you've done up till this point. Focus on all you've accomplished, not on everything you still desire to accomplish. Focus on how far you've come rather than how far you have left to go. You are amazing, and you deserve to celebrate all of you.

Journal Prompt
How would I celebrate myself every day if I was truly proud of what I've accomplished?

Day 246

Today I will accomplish everything I set my mind to.

Today, know that you are capable of anything you set your mind to. You get to choose again; you get to make it happen. The possibilities available to you are infinite. You simply need to trust and believe in that.

Journal Prompt
If you allowed yourself to do all that you truly de-

sired, what would you be doing today?

Day 247

My body is capable of anything I set my mind to.

Your body can do so much more than you give it credit for. Your body will carry you through everything that gets thrown your way. Honor it, honor you.

Journal Prompt
If you trusted that your body was capable of anything, what would you allow it to do for you?

Day 248

I will allow myself to be all of me; everybody else is taken.

Allow yourself to be you, all of you. Be authentic, stay in integrity with you, and never veer off path. You are so much more than you could ever know. Trust that.

Journal Prompt
If I trusted that I am irreplaceable and more than enough, how would that feel? How would that allow me to show up?

Day 249

I enjoy nutrient dense foods and so does my body.

Pay attention to the foods you choose. Choose nutrient dense foods rather than chemically-ridden ones. Your body and mind will thank you.

Journal Prompt
What foods am I choosing to put into my body, and how do they make me feel?

Day 250

I am radiant, and I deeply accept myself as I am.

As a radiant being, allow yourself to shine bright. Don't be shy, and don't play small. Show the world all of you because it needs you.

Journal Prompt

What would I allow myself to do today if I trusted I was needed?

Day 251

I allow my body to rest when it needs to. I honor the need for restoration.

Rest is necessary to reset. When you allow yourself some downtime to fill your cup, you are better for it. You can show up more fully for yourself and those around you. Stop doing all the time, and start allowing yourself to be.

Journal Prompt

If you allowed yourself to rest and restore, what would you be doing daily?

Part 3: Soul

Day 252

I trust the connection I have with myself, and I strengthen it every day with every choice I make.

Your connection to you is and will remain the most important connection you will ever have. Nourish it, strengthen it, and honor it.

Journal Prompt
What can I do today to connect deeply with myself?

Day 253

I am a powerful being of love and light. I get to share my gifts with the world one person at a time. I AM the change I desire to see in this world.

You get to share all that is within you with the world regardless of what that looks like. You get to be the change you wish to see because when you affect one person, in reality, you affect thousands because of the ripple effect you set forth.

Journal Prompt
If you believed your gifts needed to be shared, what would you be doing right now?

Day 254

This temple of mine is pure and vibrant. I choose to nourish it every day with positive thoughts.

Pay attention to your thoughts, and be aware of your words. The energy behind what you think and speak can be felt from across the room. Choose to focus on the good and the expansiveness that is within you.

Journal Prompt
If I stopped and paid attention to my thoughts right now, are they serving me?

Day 255

I AM aligned with my purpose, and I do things that light my soul on fire. This life is my party, and I choose to dance to my own music.

Alignment is a choice you get to make in each moment of your life. Choosing to do things that make you feel good and light your soul on fire is not selfish; it is necessary. You get to decide how your life is going to be.

Journal Prompt
If I decided to do only what is aligned for me, what would I stop doing immediately?

Day 256

The Universe is my playground.

You are the entire Universe! You get to create as you wish. You are connected to everything around you. Allow that connection to serve you on your journey.

Journal Prompt
If I believed that I was connected to everything around me, what would I be doing differently?

Day 257

I am anchored in love; therefore, infinite love streams from me, to me, and for me. I follow the divine light within to spread love wherever I go.

You were born in love. Love is the essence of who you are. Allow love to pour from you and to you, and bask in it. Allow yourself to feel unconditional love from you to you. When you become capable of that kind of love, only love will remain.

Journal Prompt
What does unconditional love mean to me?

Day 258

I am an infinite being of light. The healing energies of the Universe flow through me, to me, and for me with ease and grace.

You are an infinite being of light. You are more than the body you walk around in. You are so much more. Allow yourself to be all of who you came here to be. The healing energies of the Universe are within you; allow them to flow freely.

Journal Prompt
How do I feel knowing that healing energies are continuously flowing through me?

Day 259

I heal myself a little more each day by releasing old paradigms that have kept me shackled in fear. In healing myself, I help heal the world.

You get to release all the old and make space for the new. You are ever evolving, and in order to welcome all that serves your highest good, you must first release all that doesn't. When you let go of old limiting beliefs and fears, you allow yourself to heal on a deeper level. In healing yourself, you make space for others to heal as well.

Journal Prompt
What beliefs, fears, and stories do I get to let go of to make space for the abundance I'm calling in?

Day 260

I connect deeply with all that is pure. My higher self thrives in abundance, love, and light.

Connecting to you is the greatest gift you will ever give yourself. Embody the highest version of who you came here to be each and every day because you know you can. Allow yourself to be all of you without holding back.

Journal Prompts
What does the highest, best version of me do each day? How does he/she show up?

Day 261

I am one with me at Source, with my divine self. I am one with the Universe. I am a beautiful, radiant being.

You are one with Source because you are an extension of Source having a human experience. Let that sink in. Trust in that truth and live accordingly.

Journal Prompt
If I fully trusted that I was an extension of Source, what would I allow myself to do, to be?

Day 262

I surrender to all that I am. I honor my divinity, my purpose, and my commitments to the Universe. I am all that I am.

Surrender and when you think you're done, surrender some more because there will always be a little more to surrender. Honor yourself, and honor the light in you so that you can honor the light in others. Live your purpose every day.

Journal Prompt
If I trusted that I was a divine being with a purpose, what would I be doing?

Day 263

I am living in my truth in every moment, standing strong in my sovereignty and leaving a trail of love and light.

Stand strong in your truth, and don't deviate from your path for anyone. Stand tall in who you are; the world needs all of you, not a watered-down version trying to please everyone.

Journal Prompt
If I were fully standing in my truth, what would I no longer be available for?

Day 264

I create a ripple of high vibrational frequencies for myself and others with every thought, word, and action.

Be aware because that's where it all begins. Pay attention to the thoughts that are running through your mind over and over again. Pay attention to the words you speak silently and out loud. Pay attention to your actions and your reactions. If they are not raising your vibration, choose again.

Journal Prompt
What thoughts, words, and actions do I get to release in order to raise my vibration?

Day 265

I listen to the whispers of my soul; it is my GPS, my greatest tool to navigate this thing called life.

You have an inner compass that is desperately trying to lead the way. Are you paying attention to it? Listen to your soul; it speaks to you daily. Giving you little nudges in the direction you need to follow, showing you the lessons you are presented with, the triggers that show up, and the hurdles you get to overcome. Be aware!

Journal Prompt
If I trusted my inner compass, what do I know I need to release?

Day 266

The divine light in me honors the divine light in you. I consciously choose love and nonjudgement to be my norm.

We are all here having our own experiences and living this life. When you choose to move forward in love and to release judgement, you allow yourself and others the freedom to be yourselves. When you honor the light within you, you can honor the light in others.

Journal Prompt
If I released judgement of myself, what would I forgive myself for?

Day 267

I show up fully to share my message daily. When one person is inspired, I've created a ripple effect greater than what meets the eye.

The world needs your magic. Whatever it is you are here to do, the world needs that. Allow yourself to show up in integrity with who you are and rise to the occasion. Each person that is inspired by you will do the same, creating a massive ripple effect.

Journal Prompt
If I allowed myself to show up fully for myself and the world, what would I be doing?

Day 268

I share the messages received from my soul because I know it touches yours.

The messages you receive are meant for you, but others are most likely in need of those messages too. As we are all connected in some way, never be afraid to share your message in whatever way feels right for you. You may never know how much the world needs you right now.

Journal Prompt
If you allowed yourself to show up fully, how would you be sharing your message?

Day 269

My mission is divinely guided. I have no shame in sharing messages because I know that those who need to hear it will hear it.

Your life, your mission, and your journey are divinely guided even when you don't believe it. Every experience you live through was put on your path for your own growth and expansion and to make you stronger. Never be afraid to share what is coming through you because you would be doing a disservice to those that need what you have to share.

Journal Prompt

If I believed with every fiber of my being that my message was needed, what would I be sharing with the world?

Day 270

I follow the guidance within, knowing that whatever the outcome, it will be my most benevolent.

When you follow your inner guidance, you can never go wrong. When you listen to your heart, it will never steer you wrong whatever the outcome may be. When you trust that all is happening for your most benevolent outcome, you learn to release attachment to the outcome so that only trust remains.

Journal Prompt
If I trusted that everything is being presented to me for my most benevolent outcome and that the Universe will provide that which I desire or something better, what expectations would I let go of?

Day 271

I surrender and fall to my knees open to divine guidance not out of weakness but out of strength. This is how I rise fiercer than before.

When you surrender and come to your knees, it is

not a sign of weakness but of strength. When you bow down and surrender to the Universe, you are opening the portal of possibilities for yourself. You are telling the Universe you are ready for what it is about to send your way. You get to rise stronger than ever.

Journal Prompt
If I saw strength in my shortcomings and allowed myself to surrender, what belief would I no longer cling to?

Day 272

I sow seeds of love and light wherever I go. I am the gardener; I am the creator.

When you leave love and light in your wake, you are planting the garden of greatness. The seeds may not bloom immediately, but trust that it will eventually.

Journal Prompt
How do I contribute to this world?

Day 273

I generate my own vibration with all that I am. I choose to exist in the highest frequency and spread my light from there.

You choose your vibration with your thoughts, your words, and your actions. When you play victim and allow others to impact your mood and anything else, you are choosing a lower vibration by choosing to give your powers away. Choose wisely.

Journal Prompt

If I truly desired to exist in the highest frequency, what would I be choosing?

Day 274

I claim Sovereignty not only with my words but in the way I show up in this world. My thoughts, my actions, and my choices all stem from that state of being.

Soul Sovereignty isn't attained with words; it's attained with your energy. When you live your truth fully, stand up for what you believe in, and claim control of your life, when you live fiercely in that truth, that's when you begin to claim sovereignty. When you let go of fear and doubts, you stop allowing others to have a hold on you. When you become unwavering in who you are and what you desire, only then can you reach that level of freedom.

Journal Prompt

How do I get to show up as the Sovereign being that I am?

Day 275

I focus on connecting, healing, and growing because I'm worthy. It is not selfish; it is necessary.

Believe that you are worthy every moment of every day. Trust that you are healing and growing with every decision you make. Trust that you are releasing all that no longer serves you, all that's been holding you back. You get to live your best life; there's no need to struggle.

Journal Prompt
If I gave myself permission to be all of me and trusted that I know best, what would I no longer be available for?

Day 276

I nurture my connection with me at Source, with my divinity. There is no greater gift.

Choose to nurture your connection to you by being still, going on nature walks, and spending time with yourself to rediscover who you are. Start seeking the answers you wish to find within rather than without. You have everything you need; you simply need to allow it to come through.

Journal Prompt
What would I be doing more of if I truly desired to deepen my connection with myself?

Day 277

I tune into the soft whispers of my soul, for they never fail me. I am always divinely guided to beautiful sites within and without.

You are always divinely guided; sometimes you simply choose a different path. You will always get a nudge, a synchronicity, or a sign, but you won't always see it. Pay attention; I promise it'll be worth it.

Journal Prompt
What are some signs that I have received in the past?

Day 278

I trust my inner wisdom. I follow the guidance I receive, and I know that I am led to my destiny.

When you trust where you are led, know that the guidance within will always lead you down the most benevolent path, and all worry fades away.

Journal Prompt
If I fully trusted my inner guidance, what would I be doing right now?

Day 279

I release attachment to my old stories and programs. Today I stand strong in the knowledge that I am the quantum creator of my reality.

You are the quantum creator of your reality the moment you allow yourself to be, so trust and surrender. Feel the emotions ahead of the event. Choose to be there here and now because you can.

Journal Prompt
If I closed my eyes and found myself exactly where I desire to be, what would that look like, and more importantly, how would that feel? (Be very detailed down to the smells, the sounds, the sites, etc.)

Day 280

I consciously do things that feel unnatural so that I can become supernatural. That I am!

Make choices that scare you because you know how much they'll allow you to expand. Make decisions that aren't easy but will allow you to live fully in your truth.

Journal Prompt
What have I been holding back because of fear?

Day 281

I embody my divinity and all that it encompasses. I accept myself for who I am now.

Accept yourself for who you are, and embody the divinity within you. She/He is just sitting there waiting for you to wake up. The highest, best version of you is already here; allow him/her to shine through.

Journal Prompt
If I embodied all of me, what would that look like? How would I be showing up?

Day 282

I continue to heal each and every day for myself and for the collective.

When you heal yourself, you allow the collective to heal too. Never forget that we are all connected, and the ripple effect of your actions can be felt miles away. When you heal yourself, you're also giving those around you permission to do the same even if you never realize it.

Journal Prompt
What do I get to heal that's been buried deep inside

for years?

Day 283

I transcend all that was to step into the Divine Goddess that I am.

Choose to transcend all that you once were and all that you no longer desire to be. Choose to rise above, and step into the Divine Goddess that you are. You didn't come here to simply survive; you came here to thrive. You came here to remember the divinity within you.

Journal Prompt
How does the goddess in you desire to show up in this world?

Day 284

I honor myself for choosing to be the creator of MY path. I honor myself for trudging even when the muck gets thick. I honor myself for who I am now.

You get to choose. You get to create your own reality with every choice you make. Why would you give that power up? Release all that you've been through; it's in your past! Honor yourself for making it this far, and then decide that you get to create a new reality for yourself. One that is filled with joy and fulfillment!

Journal Prompt

How would I treat myself if I truly honored how far I've come? Where was I six months ago, and where am I now? What have I gotten through that has gotten me here?

Day 285

I am the creator but also the destroyer.

I am gentle but fierce.

I am loving but detached.

I am kind yet protective.

I exist in this duality like yin and yang.

You get to slide up and down the spectrum in order to stay in alignment with who you are. Being the best version of you and being a loving being doesn't mean you are all rainbows and unicorns. You get to be all of you and show up fully because that is what will be required of you to step up to your next level.

Journal Prompt

If I gave myself permission to be ALL that I am, what would I do now that I've been holding back on for far too long?

Day 286

I allow myself to experience the integrations that I am receiving without judgement. I am patient and kind with myself.

Allow yourself to integrate all higher aspects of you, for they complete you and allow you to be all of you.

Journal Prompt
How can I allow myself to be all of me unapologetically?

Day 287

The Universe supports my soul's desires. I create my reality with ease and grace because it's a choice that I've made.

The Universe is always striving to provide you with exactly what you desire or something better. Believe that, and trust that. When you live your life as if the Universe is conspiring in your favor because it is, there will be no doubt that everything you desire is right there waiting for you.

Journal Prompt
What is something I deeply desire that I keep telling myself all the reasons why I can't have it?

Day 288

I am always led by the Universe as I walk my path. My mission is clear, and I allow it to unfold divinely in love.

You are always led even when you don't see it. Your mission is being shown to you repeatedly; you have simply chosen not to follow your own guidance. Pay attention to all that you are being shown, and stop rationalizing all of it and trying to make it fit into a box. Allow everything that is coming through to come through.

Journal Prompt
If I knew the Universe is sending me messages every moment of every day, what old stories would I let go of?

Day 289

I am Source expressing itself in this current reality. I go where I am led and have faith that all is happening for me.

You are an extension of Source having this human experience. You came here to remember; will you allow yourself to do just that, or will you continue to fight it? Trust the process; it will pay off ten fold. Have a little faith.

Journal Prompt

If I allowed myself to be led, what would I release control of?

Day 290

I am a Sovereign being! I am love, I am light, and I am an extension of Source. I own all that I am and stand strong in the knowledge of who I am.

Step into your Sovereignty, and stop allowing everything and everyone around you to control who you are. Know what you stand for and say no to anything that isn't that!

Journal Prompt
If you were fully standing in your truth, who or what would you no longer be available for?

Day 291

I am a multidimensional being having a human experience. I release all fears and limiting beliefs, for they are not mine. I choose to be all that I am.

When you begin to realize you are a multidimensional being, you allow yourself to be all versions of you here and now. You get to release limiting beliefs and fears because they aren't yours. They are merely illusions set forth by your ego to keep you playing small. Choose to be all of you unapologetically.

Journal Prompt
Who am I without my fears and limiting beliefs?

Day 292

As I become no one, in no space nor time, I allow myself to simply be my multidimensional self.

When you allow yourself to be in the moment, to be nobody by definition, and to be nowhere but in the now, you become all that you are. If you sit in meditation and let go of your thoughts even if for just one second, you become everything and nothing all at once.

Journal Prompt
How do I feel when I sit in meditation and simply allow myself to be?

Day 293

I exist in the frequency of love. My being emanates a vibration of love. I am no longer afraid of the dark for it allows my light to shine bright.

Live in a state of unconditional love and emanate that! When you know that you are love, you become un-afraid of the dark because you know the light within you will blow that out of the water. Allow yourself to shine bright because it is your birthright.

Journal Prompt
What does unconditional love feel like?

Day 294

As I embody my Sovereign self, I choose to exist in the highest frequency.

When you show up as your sovereign self and the highest version of who you came here to be, you allow yourself to exist in a different band with, in a different frequency.

Journal Prompt
What would it look like for me to allow myself to show up as the best version of me?

Day 295

I trust my inner guidance; my compass never steers me astray. In connection to me at Source, all that comes through is pure and true.

You've left yourself bread crumbs since the moment you entered this world. It's the trail that leads to the true you. You may have ignored said trail, but it's there. You are continuously receiving messages from the Universe/ Source, showing you the next step to take and the next choice to make, but are you listening? Are you paying attention? Close your eyes and just breathe. Trust and allow your messages to come through.

Journal Prompt
Do I believe in synchronicities? Do I believe in signs?

Day 296

I make choices that are aligned with my soul's desires every waking moment. I am constantly expanding into the highest version of who I AM.

The choices you make every day are either getting you closer to your true north or farther. Making a decision that gets you farther doesn't mean failure, it means you took a right when you now know you should've taken a left. You wouldn't give up your trajectory in the car because of a wrong turn, yet in our lives we do. Choose to find your way back to the path that is you.

Journal Prompt
How would I move forward if I believed there was nothing I could fail at?

Day 297

I surrender to the powers within and allow infinite abundance to flow into my reality.

You are infinitely abundant; perhaps you've just had your blinders on. If you woke up this morning, you are abundant. If you have hot water to shower in, you are abundant. If you feel loved, you are abundant. If you can move your body however you choose to, you are abundant. If you can eat when you're hungry, you are abundant. If you feel safe, you are abundant. Abundance is in the eye of the beholder; choose to be and feel abundant.

Journal Prompt
What in my life makes me feel abundant that I perhaps have been taking for granted?

Day 298

I am the master of my reality, the master of my mind. Sovereign I stand in no space nor time.

You are the master of your life. Reclaim that now. Show up fully for the woman that you are. Choose to be all of you, no holding back. Allow yourself to let go of the labels you've been wearing so proudly and just be.

Journal Prompt
Without all the labels (wife, husband, mom, dad, daughter, son, sister, brother, friend), who are you at your core?

Day 299

I stand in my truth unwaveringly. I remain connect-ed to me and through me at Source at all times, knowing that I am unshakable.

Stand in your truth, and be unwavering in it. Do not allow anyone or anything to make you believe that you need to change. You get to be all of you, and if others are uncomfortable with that, you might want to release all that no longer supports your growth.

Journal Prompt
If I stood in my truth unwaveringly, what would I be letting go of that I've been holding onto for dear life?

Day 300

I focus on raising my vibration, for that is the one thing that is in my power. I release the desire to control any outcome because I know all unfolds as it should.

Focus on existing in the vibration of love, the vi-bration of joy, and the vibration of gratitude. Raise your vibration with each thought, word, and action. You have no control over anything but that. Let go of what you think you need to be and what you need to be doing; let it all go, and just allow all that is to be.

Journal Prompt
What can I do in this precise moment to raise my

vibration?

Day 301

I honor the warrior within me. The strength she brings, the knowing she uncovers, and the energy she emanates.

The warrior in you is strong, fierce, and confident. She/he knows how powerful she/he is, and she's/he's ready to take on the world. Are you ready?

Journal Prompt
If you allowed the warrior in you to do her/his thing, what would she/he be doing?

Day 302

I surrender to what is, knowing that it is necessary for the evolution of our collective. I lean into love and trust because something beautiful is taking place.

All happens divinely for you. Everything is happening exactly as it should; know and trust that however difficult it may be. Know that you are having the experiences necessary for your evolution. The Universe only sends your way that which will help you grow. Trust that the rainbow always comes after the storm.

Journal Prompt

Thinking back, when in your life has an experience that you may have thought was "bad" turned out to be the greatest stepping stone for you?

Day 303

As a witness and observer of the beautiful shifts happening all around me, I also recognize the magical shifts taking place within me.

The world is shifting. Are you fighting the new out of fear? Allow yourself to follow the waves of evolution, and choose to choose differently this time around. There's a new age upon us, and you get to decide who you get to be in this new age.

Journal Prompt

What changes am I fighting? Why?

Day 304

I embrace my evolution with an open heart. I learn to thrive in every situation the Universe presents me with.

When you learn to thrive through each situation you are presented with and choose to see each situation as an opportunity for growth, you'll begin to see your life through a new lens. We are only presented with what we can handle.

Journal Prompt
How can you change your perception about a current situation you are living through?

Day 305

Every cell of my body is constantly healing. Every strand of my DNA is transforming and activating. I am a multidimensional being in expansion.

Your DNA is transforming; every cell of your body is ever changing, healing, growing, and becoming more alive. With every breath you take, your entire being is evolving. Appreciate the expansion that you get to experience and continue to focus on that.

Journal Prompt
Where in the past have I not allowed myself to shift into something more?

Day 306

I am my own healer.

I am powerful.

I am unwavering.

I am all that I am!

You are exactly who you need to be in this moment, never doubt that. Know that you are your own healer; all you need is right there within you. Others can hold space for you, and they can support you, but nobody can do the work for you. Choose to stand in your power, and know that nobody can mess with you if you don't allow them to. Stand strong and sturdy in the truth of who you are.

Journal Prompt
Where have I leaned on and expected someone else to heal me?

Day 307

I shift into higher realms of consciousness with ease and flow. I choose thoughts, words, and actions that are in alignment with the frequency I desire to exist in.

The more aware you are, the more conscious you are. The higher your vibration, the more you can exist in a different bandwidth. You and you alone decide where you get to be. Remember to choose wisely.

Journal Prompt
Where do I desire to exist? What frequency do I desire to *be* in?

Day 308

I embody the highest version of the person I came here to be. I allow the essence of who I am to pour through me abundantly. I am ready to rise.

When you become so certain of who you are and begin to trust your entire being, knowing you are doing and being exactly who you came here to be, you'll allow your essence to pour from you without any fear.

Journal Prompt

Where am I holding on to an idea of who I'm supposed to be? Where do those beliefs come from?

Day 309

I trust me! I trust my intuition; I trust my inner voice. I am confident in the power of my truth.

Your intuition is real. Your guidance is pure. Your truth is exactly that.

Journal Prompt

Where in my life have I allowed myself to doubt what was coming through me? When have I known that there was something I was meant to do but simply didn't out of fear?

Day 310

I focus not on what I see but what I feel. I close my eyes and trust my divine inner compass.

Close your eyes and feel. The better you become at feeling and knowing, the easier it becomes to navigate this thing called life. What you see is merely an illusion, but what you feel is your truth.

Journal Prompt
When in your life have you chosen to ignore your feelings and your knowing and been deceived?

Day 311

I allow my consciousness to expand as I pay attention to every sound and sensation, allowing myself to lean into my experiences fully.

When you allow yourself to lean into your senses, you allow yourself to feel everything. You think less and feel more; in those moments, magic occurs.

Journal Prompt
Do I allow myself to feel more, or am I stuck in my head? How do I get to change that?

Day 312

I allow my soul to lead the way, listening to every whisper, paying attention to every synchronicity, and seeing all the signs.

When you become open to receiving without expectation and trust the Universe and pay attention to all the subtle signs, you begin to see a clearer picture. Allow yourself to be guided by the highest version of you; the one who already knows how it all goes.

Journal Prompt
Where in my life am I being resistant? Where can I let go of my expectations and allow life to unfold?

Day 313

The Universe speaks to me, and I listen. The subtle synchronicities need not go unseen. The messages are received with love and gratitude.

Be open to all the Universe is whispering in your ear. Open your heart, and be ready to receive in every moment of every day. Allow abundance to flow to you with ease and grace.

Journal Prompt
Where has the Universe showered me with abundance today?

Day 314

I allow myself space to heal daily.

Trust that all is happening as it should. Your past has led you to this space in time. The work you've done this far has prepared you for the deeper healing you get to do. Give yourself space to do the work, and honor yourself while you heal generations of hurt.

Journal Prompt
What do I get to heal today?

Day 315

I continuously bring myself back into alignment. It's how I get to grow.

When you find yourself saying yes to things your soul is screaming no to, and find yourself thinking thoughts that don't serve you, and speaking words out of anger, you are not in alignment. In that moment, you catch yourself, shift, and come back to center. That's how you get to grow.

Journal Prompt
What is a thought that no longer serves me that I get to shift out of?

Day 316

I choose to sit in silence when the world seems to be in chaos.

Regardless of what's happening in the world around you, you always have a choice to choose inner peace. It's a choice. You must understand that when you allow the chaos to seep in, you're allowing everything and everyone around you control of your being. You can have compassion while still honoring your peace. You can empathize while protecting your energy. When we sit in stillness and calm our world, we create a ripple effect in the collective; you get to do your part.

Journal Prompt
Where in my life have I been allowing the outer chaos to affect my inner peace? How do I get to change that?

Day 317

I deepen my connection to self with every breath I consciously take.

Every breath you take is life. Every conscious breath you take allows you to deepen your connection to self. When you are able to lose yourself in the rhythm of your breath and the rhythm of your heartbeat, you become it. So right here, right now, be conscious of your breath, close your eyes, and surrender to it.

Journal Prompt
How does it feel when I simply flow with my breath?

Day 318

I must demolish the old to create space for the new.

You get to release the old to make space for the new in all areas of your life. You get to say no to all that insults your soul so that you can say yes to all that lights it up. You get to let go of people that have been holding you back to make space in your circle for those that will lift you up. You get to focus on creating space in your thoughts, within your words, your actions, and your reactions for all that serves your highest good.

Journal Prompt
Where have I not been impeccable with my words, thoughts, actions, and reactions today? How can I change that?

Day 319

I connect to my heart because from there I can feel the truth.

Your heart always knows best. Your heart is your true north, your "brain." Connect to that space within you, and allow it to expand. In that space you can find your truth.

Journal Prompt
If I close my eyes and connect to my heart space, what do I feel?

Day 320

I get to be the objective observer of my life, allowing all that arises to come and go.

When you can take a step back and see your life as it is through the lens of neutrality without the charged emotions, you can easily detach from any outcome. When you know that all is happening FOR you, you can lean into trust, and allow life to come and go with ease and flow.

Journal Prompt
If I fully trusted that all is happening FOR me and not TO me, what beliefs could I let go of?

Day 321

My soul dances to the rhythm of its own tune.

Allow yourself to find your own rhythm and start dancing to your own beat. We are all unique individuals here having a unique experience. Trust that with your entire being.

Journal Prompt
What does my soul desire to do today?

Day 322

I allow myself to tune into the vibrations of the Universe to become in harmony with everything around me.

When we tune in, we can find the frequency that feels good to us. We can block any and all lower vibrations, and protect our energy to stay high vibe. Close your eyes and feel.

Journal Prompt
How would it feel to tune into a higher vibration right now?

Day 323

I peel back the layers of my existence, allowing myself to connect back to the core of who I am.

When you allow yourself to peel back the layers that no longer serve you, you begin to step into who you were always meant to be. In this moment right now, you get to be her/him, all of her/him.

Journal Prompt

What are some old beliefs and programs that I choose to let go of right here and now?

Day 324

I release the pain and suffering from this lifetime and past ones so that I can move forward with strength.

Choose to let go of all trauma even that which you may not fully remember. Set the intention to move forward each day with a higher level of consciousness. Choose to release all that no longer serves you so that you can move forward without unnecessary baggage.

Journal Prompt

What pain have I been holding onto like a badge of honor that I now get to release?

Day 325

I transcend my fears to create more space for surrender.

When you choose to transmute and transcend your fears, you are surrendering. Fears are but an illusion, ones we get to dismantle for our greater good.

Journal Prompt

What fears have I been allowing to hold me back? How can I find proof that this fear is not real?

Day 326

I am no longer available to be affected by other energies. I am protected. I am safe.

When you leave yourself open to absorb other energy, you leave yourself open to feel all sorts of ways. You get to protect your energy because it is sacred. Stop allowing others moods, words, or actions affect the way you feel. Reclaim control!

Journal Prompt
When do I typically allow others to affect me? What do I choose moving forward?

Day 327

I am a spiritual being having a fabulous human experience. I choose to embrace all of it.

Embrace this experience you're having, and know that you chose this even if you don't remember. When you stop resisting and begin embracing all that is taking place, life begins to look a lot different.

Journal Prompt

What is something I could've embraced today if I had chosen to change my perspective?

Day 328

I cannot be created or destroyed; I can merely be transmuted.

Trust that transmutation is the only true occurrence. When you move forward with this knowing, life as you know it will not be the same.

Journal Prompt
If I fully trusted that all is transmuted, how would I move forward today?

Day 329

I am not this body; I am this spirit. I am all that I am.

Your body is merely the "suit" that allows you to have this human experience; the true essence of who you are is your spirit, your soul. Choose to be all of you un-apologetically because it's your birthright!

Journal Prompt
If I no longer defined myself with my body, who would I be?

Day 330

I dive deeper into the truth of who I am with every meditation.

When we meditate, we allow our minds to become still even if it's just for a millisecond. Those milliseconds are where the magic happens; those are the moments you access zero point. When you can become no one, in no time nor space, in that moment, you are simply all that you are.

Journal Prompt
How can I tune into ME even more?

Day 331

I focus on the energy that allows me to expand and release all energies that seek to contract.

They say wherever your attention goes, your energy goes. They also say that whatever you focus on expands. It's imperative that you choose what you focus your attention on wisely.

Journal Prompt
What are the things that I have been focusing on that feel constrictive? What can I choose to focus on instead?

Day 332

I allow myself to release everything that I am not, so that I can fully step into everything that I am.

When you consciously choose to no longer carry around the illusions of who you are and remove the mask, you allow yourself to fully step into who you were always meant to be. Do not judge the mask as it once upon a time served you. Now that it does not serve you, feel how freeing it is to finally leave it behind.

Journal Prompt
What are aspects of me that no longer serve me do I get to leave behind?

Day 333

As I raise my awareness, I no longer seek to control the outcome but rather wish for the most benevolent outcome.

We often tend to wish for a certain outcome for ourselves and others. The problem with that is that we have no idea what is in someone else's best interest. Allow yourself to simply wish for the most benevolent outcome for all even if you don't understand it all.

Journal Prompt
If I fully trusted that all unfolds as it should, what would I change in my life?

Day 334

I now seek within the answers I spent years seeking without.

You have always had the answers within you; you simply didn't know it. We often seek answers from others, but remember that nobody can know YOU as well as you do. Nobody can understand what is in your best interest but you. So tune into YOU, and seek your answers there because that's how you'll never be steered astray!

Journal Prompt
When in my life have I sought out answers from others? How can I tune into me and trust me more?

Day 335

I am an infinite source of light; I allow myself to shine bright enough to allow others to find theirs.

You are the light, and when you allow yourself to shine bright, you light the path that allows others to do the same. We have no idea how massive of an impact we have, so always BE as if all eyes were on you!

Journal Prompt
How do I get to let my light shine through even more today?

Day 336

I converse with the Universe in frequency, not words.

The Universe speaks frequency, not words. When you say you desire one thing, but your thoughts are that you are not worthy of those things or that you can never have them, your energy backs those thoughts up, and that's what the Universe picks up on. So rather than speaking with words, change your frequency!

Journal Prompt
Where have I been sending the Universe the wrong message?

Day 337

I surround myself with like-minded beings within the same frequency.

Choose to surround yourself by those who vibrate equal to you or higher. It has been said that we are represented by the five people we are closest to. If you look around, what does that say about you? Make sure you're pleased with the answer to that question.

Journal Prompt
Who in your circle does not support your growth and expansion? Reflect upon that for a moment.

Day 338

I live in harmony with those I allow into my circle. I am no longer available for small talk and chaos.

When you begin to "spring clean" your friends list in reality and virtually, you will feel so much better. When you allow people to bring chaos, stress, and anxiety into your life, you are basically allowing them to walk through your mind with their dirty feet, and then you have to clean up the mess! Choose to focus on those that lift you up, and choose those with which you can have meaningful conversations. It's not selfish; it's necessary for your wellbeing!

Journal Prompt
How would my circle be different if I were no longer available for anyone that dragged me down?

Day 339

I am a unique being here to have a unique experience. I am in competition with no one but the version of me I was yesterday.

You didn't come here to be better than anybody but the version of you from yesterday. You see, you'll never be anybody but you, and why would you want to be? Focus on stepping more into YOU each and every day. Focus on living your happiest and healthiest life each and every day; that's what this is all about.

Journal Prompt

What can I do today to be happier and healthier than yesterday?

Day 340

I am open to receive the messages I am ready to comprehend.

Sometimes we want to know it all now. We ask for messages or answers to be shown to us, yet we're not truly ready for the answer to be delivered. Rather than asking for something you're not quite ready for, how about you trust the process? How about you allow all to arise as it should. Start paying attention to all the little things too because often times the answers don't come the way we think they will!

Journal Prompt
What are the small gifts or synchronicities that presented themselves to me today?

Day 341

All possibilities are available to me in this moment. I am open for each and every one that will help me expand into the being I was always meant to be.

There are infinite possibilities available to us in each and every moment we simply don't allow. When we trust that everything is possible and that it's all there for the taking, we start being different, living differently. Trust the process and become open to receive.

Journal Prompt
What is something that I deeply desire, yet don't believe I'm capable of having?

Day 342

I seek the divine in you as I seek the divine in me.

Always be on the lookout for the divine in you and others. When you show up in your divinity, you allow others to do the same.

Journal Prompt
How do I allow the divine in me to shine through?

Day 343

I am awake for the beautiful unfolding that is taking place.

So many spend their lives on auto pilot, missing all

the little things in life, which are in fact the big things. So many continuously strive for more: more material, more money, and more "things" they think will bring them joy, yet they miss out on the beauty that surrounds them. They're so focused on the past or the future that they miss every now moment they were meant to enjoy. Don't be that person!

Journal Prompt

How can I be more present today to enjoy the gifts life is continuously showering me with?

Day 344

I release all harmful energies from my being and allow my light to transmute them.

When you focus on your light and its powers, you can transmute anything that isn't in your highest good. Let go of less benevolent energies and send them off with love. Tune into your loving light and allow it to permeate your entire being, leaving no space for anything else.

Journal Prompt

What are some energies that no longer serve me that I get to transmute?

Day 345

I embrace the benevolent flow of transcendence that occurs within me and without.

Transcendence is a beautiful thing. Allow it to take place without resistance. Allow all to unfold exactly as it should; let go of the reins.

Journal Prompt
How can I allow more flow in my life?

Day 346

I surrender to all that is, and then I surrender a little more.

There will always be more surrendering to be done. This journey is one of surrendering over and over again. Choosing to let go of all that we thought we needed to be, all that we believed to know. It's about knowing that the Universe always has a safety net ready to catch you.

Journal Prompt
What is an outcome I've been desperately trying to control that I now get to surrender?

Day 347

Paradise isn't a place; it's a state of being.

We often think that paradise is a place somewhere tropical, somewhere we'd want to go on vacation. When you shift your perspective and you embrace the fact that YOU are your own paradise, there's no more seeking because wherever you are becomes paradise!

Journal Prompt
How does paradise or the idea of paradise make me feel?

Day 348

I release every version of me that got me to who I am today. I needed them then, but I no longer need them now.

Every version of you along the way was necessary to get you where you are in this moment. You no longer need them though! You are stepping more into the highest version of you every day, so embrace that.

Journal Prompt
What is a belief you've had for years? How old were you when you first remember thinking that? With the knowledge you have now, is that belief still true?

Day 349

I choose to raise my vibration regardless of anything

going on around me, for my energy is contagious.

Choose to raise your vibration regardless of what may be happening around you. You can do that by focusing on gratitude, things, people, or places that bring you joy. Giving back always helps us feel good and raise our vibration. Do things that are in alignment with who you are. Know that when you raise your vibration, there's a ripple effect that affects every person you come into contact with.

Journal Prompt
How do I get to raise my vibration consciously today?

Day 350

I am part of the cosmos. I am part of the Universe. I am part of everything and everyone.

We all come from the Universe; we're part of the cosmos. Each and every one of us is an intricate part of this system we exist in. Pay attention to how you treat yourself, how you treat others. Never doubt how important you are!

Journal Prompt
If you truly believed we are all part of the same whole, what would you be doing differently each and every day?

Day 351

I am in a continuous state of transmutation, releasing the old and creating the new.

Every day we are evolving, changing, and transmuting the old to make space for the new. Our organs, thoughts, and tastes are regenerating each day. Change is inevitable, but growth is optional, so pay attention and make sure that you are growing and evolving in the process.

Journal Prompt
How am I different than the person I was six months ago?

Day 352

I am my own religion. I am my own compass. I am all that I am.

You are all that you need. You have everything required to live within you. You are truly your own internal compass. You know what's best for you; you simply choose to not pay attention more than you'd like to admit. Change that because you can. Start paying attention to what your heart is guiding you to do. Pay attention to the signs and synchronicities that are handed to you.

Journal Prompt
If I fully trusted my intuition, my inner compass,

what is something I would've done differently this month?

Day 353

I focus on emanating the energy of that which I desire.

We know the Universe speaks frequency, and we know that everything is energy and that what you put out you also call in. If you desire to be happy, stop focusing on the fact that you need "something" more to be happy, and be happy already. If you desire to feel successful, close your eyes and imagine what your success feels like, and feel that now. If you want to be healthy, make choices that are in alignment with that. Stop focusing on all the things you don't, and focus on you already being that.

Journal Prompt
What is it that I deeply desire, and how will I feel when I get it?

Day 354

Every day I choose to take soul aligned action to make my dreams come true.

Making your dreams come true won't happen over

night. It will take dedication, commitment, and a lot of aligned action. You'll get to put your energy where your mouth is and create your dreams into reality because you can. You must believe without an ounce of doubt that you get to be and have what your soul desires or the Universe will provide you with something better.

Journal Prompt
What do you get to decide you want, and how do you get to take aligned action now to make that come true?

Day 355

I am pure consciousness.

You are pure consciousness. You've simply forgotten. Close your eyes and tune in. Quiet your mind without judgement, and meditate, move your body. Sit with yourself and pay attention.

Journal Prompt
What have I noticed while focusing on being more conscious?

Day 356

I activate and reprogram my DNA for the experiences I am meant to have.

We all have dormant DNA, and it gets to be activated. You get to take on the task of waking up to all that you are in order to do so. Once activated, you will begin to notice shifts in ways you never thought possible.

Journal Prompt

What would it mean for me to activate new strands of DNA?

Day 357

I am always exactly where I need to be.

Trust that you are always exactly where you need to be in each and every moment. Never have regrets. Always pay attention to the lessons you've learned and the knowledge you've gained. There's a lesson in everything we go through even if we can't see it in the moment. There's always something way bigger than meets the eye. Pay attention, shift your perception, and look for the lesson, for when you seek the lesson, you'll never see failure.

Journal Prompt

How would I feel if I knew and trusted that I was always exactly where I was meant to be each and every moment of my life?

Day 358

I allow myself to be open to receive. I release all fears and judgements of who I am.

When you release judgement of who you are and let go of your fears, you open yourself up to all the possibilities available to you. When you allow yourself to receive openly without expectation, you allow abundance to flow to you. Know that nothing you do is good or bad; it just is. "Good" and "bad" are qualitative words we've been taught to use since a young age. They are words that shouldn't exist because what may be good for one may not be for all. It always comes down to perception, past experiences, and knowledge. So just be and watch how life unfolds.

Journal Prompt

Where in my life have I allowed judgement of myself and my fears to hold me back? What is a new belief I choose to lean into around this?

Day 359

I cleanse my energetic field in order to remain protected in my space of alignment.

When you cleanse and protect your energy, you ensure that your space remains sacred. It's like wearing a seatbelt or brushing your teeth. It's a great way to prevent any mishaps. Protect your energy at all costs because it's worth it.

Journal Prompt

When in the past have I walked into the room and suddenly felt something off, a heaviness? How did that make me feel?

Day 360

My existence is exactly as it should be, and I embrace all of it.

We tend to always want something different, something more, when once upon a time we wished for exactly what we have in this moment. It puts things into perspective a bit, doesn't it? Embrace all that you are and all that you have because it's here, now. There is no other moment than the now. When you continuously strive for more, you miss all the beauties of in your now.

Journal Prompt

Was there a time in my life when I wished for what I have now? Back then, how did I believe I would feel once I'd accomplished that?

Day 361

I choose to expand into a higher frequency for me and for everyone around me.

Higher consciousness is a choice. Raising your frequency is a choice. One that no one can make or take away from you. When you raise your vibration, you raise the vibration of the collective. When you are happy, your happiness can be felt by those around you because your energy presents you before you walk into a room. The same goes for when you're grumpy. So before you walk into a room with other people, check in and see where your energy is at, and notice how it affects those around you.

Journal Prompt
What would I be doing differently if I knew beyond a doubt that my energy affected those around me?

Day 362

I am greater than my body, and I am greater than my mind. I am pure consciousness, and that is my superpower.

You're not your body, and you're not your mind. You are a soul having a human experience; you are pure consciousness. Stop giving yourself all these labels that mean nothing at the end of the day. Learn to love yourself unconditionally because that's what you get to do. The standards we try to exceed were taught by society and by the programs we've been instilled with since birth. You are greater than anything measurable. You are YOU, and that is a beautiful thing; it's something to celebrate.

Journal Prompt

How do I get to love myself unconditionally from this moment forward?

Day 363

I trust the frequencies that are poured down on me, and I allow them to permeate my being.

Frequencies are always being poured down from the ethers. Maybe you feel them, maybe you don't, but they're there. This might explain some sensations you've felt in the past. Always set the intention to receive only that which is sanctioned by you at Source, and trust that that is exactly what will occur. Trust that the energies you are receiving are for your most benevolent outcome.

Journal Prompt

How would it feel to know that everything is happening for you, truly?

Day 364

I focus on the energy emanated by those around me, not on their words.

Focus on the energy people are putting out, not their words. Pay attention to their behavior. Pay attention to how they treat you and others. Never ever trust words.

Journal Prompt

Who in my life have I trusted based upon the words they spoke to realize I shouldn't have? How did that make me feel?

Day 365

I create a magical experience for myself because I align wholeheartedly with that possibility.

When you stay open to the possibility that every day is a miracle and that magical experiences await you, that's what you get to create into reality. That doesn't mean you'll walk out the door and a brand new car will have appeared. It means that you should be on the look-out for the small miracles just as much as the big ones.

Journal Prompt

What are some magical moments that I've taken for granted?

I hope this book will have been a powerful tool that you will continue to dive into each and every day. Our work is never done and I for one will continue to seek growth and expansion in every way possible. I am here for the journey of becoming. These affirmations and journal prompts are meant to help elevate your spirit, raise your frequency and allow you to tap into a higher vibration on the daily. My hope is that it has done just that and will continue to do so.

Author Bio

Jen is a certified Holistic Health Coach who helps her clients become crystal clear on their desires, remove toxicity and blocks from all areas of their lives, and finally start living a life of freedom. She combines her expertise in holistic health, mindset work, and energy healing to ensure her clients fully embody these shifts. Jen is a firm believer that in order to live your best life now, you need to align, mind, body and soul.

She's certified through the Institute for Integrative Nutrition as well as a certified Advanced Marconics Practitioner, trained by the founder herself, Alison David-Bird (energy healing modality). Marconics is a powerful energy healing modality that allows the client to raise their vibration above the frequency of fear that has shackled them to their story.

She's been a guest at several womens summits and podcasts and featured in Thrive Global, The Elephant Journal as well as Sivana East. She writes regularly at www.jengagnon.rocks/blog